The Keto Effect for Woman

Stop Sugar Cravings, Reset Your Hormones and Lose Fat Fast With The Ketogenic Diet

ISBN 978-0-6486577-1-2

Michael Zollo

Table of Contents

Free Report , The 7 Keto foods you need to avoid

As a thank you for choosing my book I'd like to offer you a free report I have which talks about **the 6 Keto Foods you need to avoid** in order to make this journey as healthy and as successful as possible

On top of this I will tell you about **the 4 popular diet tips you should NEVER follow**.

Just go to www.vipketoreport.com and I will send it straight to your inbox

I would also like to invite you to join my private Facebook community for extra support and guidance

Simply type in Keto conquer 101; learn to win the weight loss game into the facebook search engine and request to join

Also follow me on Instagram at **effortless_weightloss**

Any questions, feel free to email me at **michael.zollo@hotmail.com**

Introduction

Today, nearly everyone has tried out one diet or another, hoping to lose weight or to cleanse out their system. In most cases, the word diet has been associated with starvation, moodiness, and unhealthy eating. It is generally characterized as a fad. Worse still, some people have found themselves gaining weight while on a diet that was supposed to help them lose weight. All this can be quite frustrating. It is, therefore, no wonder that some people have given up on dieting, forgetting that the weight-loss journey is a three-part process that involves physical exercise, a positive mindset, and a diet!

However, I am truly glad that you have decided to read this book as it will introduce you to everything that you need to know about the ketogenic diet. It could be that you just want to learn what the ketogenic diet is or you could actually be interested in picking up the ketogenic diet for weight loss. Whatever the reason, I am glad that you have picked up this book. I am sure you will not regret it!

Throughout this book, you will learn that the ketogenic diet is not merely a diet but a lifestyle change that will provide your body with a myriad of benefits for your health and general well-being. This implies that there are so many benefits that you will expect to reap from the ketogenic diet, aside from weight loss.

As you begin your journey, it is important for you to know that the ketogenic diet goes by a few names, depending on the context. By far, the most popular name for the diet is its shortened form, keto. People also refer to the diet as the Low Carb-High Fat (LCHF) diet or the Very Low Carb Diet (VLCD).

Despite the many names that may be used to refer to the diet, the underlying concept remains the same, which is getting your body into the state of ketosis.

If you are a complete beginner and have never heard of the concept of the ketogenic diet, worry not. This book will give you a step-by-step guide to build your understanding of the ketogenic diet and hopefully get you excited about it. For many beginners, it may sound counter-intuitive to use a high-fat diet to lose weight. However, I do assure you that by the end of this book, you will come to fully appreciate the concept of ketosis.

While there is scientific research that has proven the long-term benefits of the ketogenic diet to your weight and overall health, many women still shy away from the diet due to the negative publicity that has long been done by the press. However, I promise you that if you stick to this book, you will come to fully comprehend how it is that the ketogenic diet applies to women. You will come to appreciate some of the female specific benefits which go a long way in improving your health and well-being.

If you are an older woman approaching menopause, do not get worried, we've got you covered. This book will expound on the challenges that pre-menopausal, menopausal, and post-menopausal women go through and some of the ways in which the ketogenic diet could alleviate some of the signs and symptoms of menopause.

While there are many factors that cause obesity, it is scientifically proven that obesity is hormonal and not a result of a caloric imbalance or excessive consumption of calories. When we eat, the food is broken down and converted into glucose, which is a source of energy for the body. Insulin is a hormone that is involved in the absorption of glucose and the storage of excess glucose as fats. Hence, it causes cells in the body to absorb this glucose for energy. However, when we eat excessively, the insulin in the bloodstream increases, signaling the body to store most of this glucose as fat, contributing to obesity and weight gain.

Having seen that the hormone insulin is responsible for most cases of obesity, the natural solution is to find ways that will reduce the amount of insulin in the bloodstream. Two of the most common ways of reducing insulin levels in the bloodstream are the ketogenic diet and the intermittent fasting diet.

In this book, we focus on the ketogenic diet, a high-fat, moderate-protein, and low-carb diet that force the body into a state of ketosis. During ketosis, the body breaks down the fats in the body to release energy. The breakdown of fats eventually leads to significant weight loss.

It is arguable that the most important aspect of the ketogenic diet is developing the discipline and will power to stick to the diet, despite the intense cravings that people experience. This is because cravings are a powerful feeling that can de-motivate and disorient you. In some cases, some people are completely unable to focus on their day-to-day activities due to the intense cravings they experience.

Many people cite that the most difficult aspect of the ketogenic diet is not the cravings that you will experience, but instead, it is the sheer determination that it will take for you to avoid the conventional foods that are highly processed and rich in fats. As such, the main reason why the ketogenic diet fails is that people give in to their bodily urges and social demands in relation to food. Inconsistency and the inability to follow through with your caloric restrictions will set you up for failure.

Due to the somewhat extreme nature of the ketogenic diet, it is not recommended for all people. If you are known to have a history of an eating disorder or are underweight, this diet is may not be for you. Pregnant and lactating women too should avoid this diet. All women should carefully approach this diet as there are instances where it interferes with the natural menstrual cycle. People who suffer from type 2 diabetes or any other medical conditions should also approach the diet with caution. Generally, it is highly recommended that you seek the advice of a medical practitioner before starting the diet.

In this book, we aim to provide conclusive knowledge of the ketogenic diet, while clarifying some of the myths and misconceptions that are often related to this topic. With that in mind, I would like to wish you happy reading! May you find a way to apply the lessons learnt from this book, if not to your life, then to the life of a loved one.

Chapter 1: What is the Ketogenic Diet?

The Science behind the Diet

You've probably heard of the phrase 'keto diet' used among fitness experts and other individuals looking to hit their fitness goals. This is because, in the recent past, people have been very excited about the ketogenic diet, seeing it as one of the most popular ways to shed off a few extra kilos. In addition, medical practitioners and nutritionists from across the globe have reported an increase in the number of inquiries on the ketogenic diet. However, if you have not heard about it, worry not, this book is just for you!

The ketogenic diet is a high-fat, moderate-protein, and low-carbohydrate diet that has been proven to have a myriad of benefits for your health and general body performance. The diet derives its name from the word 'ketosis,' a natural metabolic state of the body in which the body breaks down fat stored in the body to release ketone molecules. Ketones are an alternative source of energy which can provide the entire body with the energy that is needed for normal functioning.

Under normal circumstances, the cells in the body use glucose as the primary source of energy. Glucose is derived whenever the body breaks down dietary carbohydrates such as starch and sugars found in other foods. The body then breaks down the carbohydrates into simple sugars such as glucose. Glucose is either broken down to release energy or stored in the liver in the form of glycogen.

In the absence of sufficient glucose to meet the body's energy demands, the body will adapt an alternative strategy to ensure its proper functioning. Specifically, the liver breaks down fat reserves in the body into fatty acids and ketone bodies. The ketone bodies are then passed into the bloodstream, replacing glucose as a source of energy. As such, the body burns fats rather than carbohydrates to produce energy, and this state is known as ketosis.

The History of the Ketogenic Diet

Despite the recent hype, the diet ketogenic has been used by medical experts for more than one hundred years. It was initially popularized in the early 1920s and 1930s as a dietary therapy for epileptic patients, which also served as an alternative treatment. Today, the diet has proven benefits for weight loss, and the general health and performance of epileptic and diabetic patients.

The ketogenic diet has its roots in the ancient practice of fasting, and other dietary regimes that were used as a treatment for epilepsy. These ancient practices were used from as early as 500 B.C., in the days of the ancient Greeks. These treatments included the excess or limitation of some animal, plant, or mineral substances.

In the early 1920s, modern physicians began to mimic the biochemical effects of fasting and starvation to treat epilepsy. A pair of French physicians, (Guelpa & Marie, 1911) were the first to record the use of starvation as a treatment for epilepsy. The pair treated 20 children and adults and reported that the seizures were less during the treatment period. For the next two decades, physicians and medical doctors conducted wide-spread research and tests on this method of treatment, during which the method was widely used.

In 1921 specifically, an endocrinologist known as Dr. Rollin Woodyatt observed that three compounds (today known as ketone bodies) were produced in the liver as a result of fasting or feeding on a low-carb, high-protein diet. It was in the same year that Russell Wilder from the Mayo clinic termed it as the 'ketogenic diet' and used it for the treatment of epilepsy.

However, the use of the diet declined in the late 1930s after the discovery of anti-convulsant drugs and therapies. Once the anti-convulsant drugs rose in popularity, doctors were no longer trained on the ketogenic diet. As such, the few doctors who tried to implement this treatment failed to achieve the desired results. This is because, for optimal results with the ketogenic diet, it is important to follow it properly as required to stimulate the production and release of ketone molecules.

In the 1970s, the ketogenic diet once again rose in popularity due to its effect on weight loss. A very low carbohydrate diet for weight loss was popularized by Dr. Atkins in his paper (Atkins, 1972). The diet began with a two-week ketogenic phase that allowed for zero intake of carbohydrates. This was followed by gradual addition of carbohydrates that ensured that the body kept burning its fat as fuel. Hence, individuals would continue to lose without hunger.

How does Ketosis Work?

Food is the main source of energy for the body. This energy is supplied by three main nutrients which are carbohydrates, fats, and proteins. Hence, whenever you consume any food, the body will typically break down the carbohydrates first followed by the fats and the proteins.

Under normal circumstances, the body's functionality primarily relies on carbohydrates as a source of fuel. The carbohydrates are then usually broken down into glucose, which is the primary source of energy for the body. Despite glucose being the primary source of energy for the body, it is not the only way that our body can get energy for its proper functioning.

Ketosis is a natural metabolic state that occurs whenever your intake of carbohydrates is low. This, in turn, leads to a decrease in the supply of glucose within the bloodstream. To ensure the proper functioning of the body, the body will need to find an alternative source of fuel.

Whenever you fast or take part in the ketogenic diet, you significantly reduce the amount of carbohydrates that you are consuming and consequently you limit the amount of glucose produced by the body. The decrease in the glucose levels in the bloodstream triggers the metabolic state of ketosis where fat is used as an alternative source of fuel.

The state of ketosis is characterized by the breakdown of fats stored in the adipose tissue and ketogenic amino acids to release ketone bodies, which are also known as ketones. The ketone bodies then float within the bloodstream, supplying energy to the body cells and organs.

The ketogenic diet primarily relies on the breakdown of fats to release energy for the body. When used consistently, the body and brain will now rely on the breakdown of fats to release ketone bodies which are a source of energy. This implies that the body will begin to burn down and utilize the stored fat, eventually leading to weight loss.

The body can take anywhere from a couple of days to weeks to fully attain the state of ketosis. It generally varies from one person to the next. Once the body has fully entered into the state of ketosis, you will expect a decrease in the production of glucose and an increase in the breakdown of fats to produce energy for the body. There are some specific symptoms that you will need to look out for to confirm that your body has fully entered the state of ketosis. You will, therefore, need to consistently monitor your body as you begin your ketogenic diet journey.

The Relationship between the Ketogenic Diet and Ketosis

As mentioned earlier, the ketogenic diet is a high-fat, moderate-protein, and low-carb diet. The diet reduces the amount of carbohydrates consumed, replacing them with healthy fats. The decrease in carbohydrates consequently leads to a decrease in glucose, forcing the body into a state of ketosis where it utilizes fat as an alternative source of energy.

While on this diet, you will typically obtain 75% of your daily nutrient requirements from fats, 20% from protein, and 5% from carbohydrates. In addition to reducing your intake of carbohydrates, the diet also focuses on eating less processed foods and more real, healthy, and organic foods.

Types of Ketogenic Diets

There are different ways in which people approach the ketogenic diet. So far, there are 4 types which are widely accepted and used around the world.

The Standard Ketogenic Diet (SKD) is a diet that contains all the classic macronutrients in specified portions. 75% of the diet contains fat, 20% protein, and 5% carbohydrates. As such, it is a high-fat, moderate-protein, and low-carb diet. It is the most widely used type of ketogenic diet.

The Targeted Ketogenic Diet (TKD) allows people to add the amount of carbohydrates that they can consume only during the periods before and after a workout. This ensures that any carbohydrates that are consumed are actually burnt down during exercise.

The Cyclical Ketogenic Diet (CKD) involves going in and out of ketosis during planned intervals such that it becomes cyclical. It could involve 5 days of a ketogenic diet followed by 2 days of high-carb feeding. There could also be many other variations to this type of ketogenic dieting.

The High-Protein Ketogenic Diet (HKD) is similar to the Standard Ketogenic Diet, the only difference being that it involves more proteins. The diet typically contains 60% fat, 35% protein, and 5% carbohydrates.

Signs and Symptoms of Ketosis

So far, you know what the ketogenic diet is and how it came into being. The next thing you need to familiarize yourself with is how to know that your body is in a state of ketosis. As aforementioned, ketosis is the process by which the body breaks down the fat stored in the body to produce ketone bodies which in turn provide the body with energy to support normal functioning.

The body will take anywhere from three days to a week to fully enter the state of ketosis. It typically varies from one person to the next and entirely depends on how you ease yourself into the ketogenic diet. There are some signs and symptoms that you could look out for to help you understand whether your body is in the state of ketosis and if not, the body's progress in the change from using glucose to ketone bodies for energy.

One of the ways in which you can determine whether your body has entered the state of ketosis is to check the level of ketone bodies in your bloodstream. This is usually achieved by using a urine test or a blood sugar meter, both of which should be able to measure ketones. These kits can be picked up at your local drug store. As such, there is no need to visit a doctor.

When the ketone levels in the body increase significantly such that some of them are not useful, they are usually excreted through urine. As such, you could use a urine strip which will measure the excess amounts of ketones in your body. While the test may be easy, it does not provide reliable results especially when an individual is well hydrated.

A breath meter or analyzer could also be used to determine whether or not your body has achieved the state of ketosis. Acetone refers to a specific ketone body that is usually released during the state of ketosis. The meter usually detects the amount of acetone in your breathe to determine the progress of the state of ketosis in your body. While it is the most affordable method, it is the least reliable method.

Blood testing, though expensive, is the most reliable method that is used to determine the ketone levels in your body. It involves lightly pricking your finger and squeezing a drop of blood on to a test kit to determine the amount of Beta-Hydroxybutyrate that is present in your blood. Like acetone, Beta-Hydroxybutyrate is a ketone body that is released during ketosis.

While carrying out the tests, you should be aware that the normal level of ketones in the bloodstream is usually 0.6 millimoles per liter. Any level above this is usually a sign of ketosis.

On the other hand, people could look out for specific signs and symptoms to determine whether or not their bodies are in the state of ketosis. One of the most common signs that you have achieved full ketosis is the occurrence of bad breath. Many people report experiencing a bad or fruity smell whenever they start the ketogenic diet. As disgusting as this may sound, it is a good sign that your body has achieved the state of ketosis.

The bad or fruity smell is usually caused by acetone. Acetone is a ketone body that exists in your breath and urine whenever your body is in the state of ketosis. Elevated levels of ketones are usually responsible for the bad or fruity smell that people experience.

To avoid walking around and speaking to people while your mouth is stinking, people usually brush their teeth regularly in the course of the day. Alternatively, you could use sugar-free gum or mint to keep your breath fresh at all times. When selecting your gum of choice, you should always look out for and avoid any that are loaded with carbohydrates. Carbohydrates will only serve to slow down the state of ketosis in your body.

Another sign that your body has achieved the state of ketosis is weight loss. Like other low-carb diets, the ketogenic diet is very efficient in helping you to shed off a few extra pounds. It is especially preferred to other diets because it ensures that you do not regain the weight that you have lost. As such, the weight loss is both short term and long term.

Most people will experience significant weight loss within the first week. While many people believe that this is fat-loss, it has scientifically been proven to be the breakdown of stored carbohydrates and water being used up. After the first week or so, the weight loss will become more consistent as long as you stick to the ketogenic diet and maintain a caloric deficit. It must, however, be noted that weight loss only occurs when you follow the ketogenic diet program.

Following a strict ketogenic diet has also been scientifically proven to result in hunger and appetite suppression. While this is still being investigated by scientists, it is believed that the elevated ketones in the body suppress the production of the ghrelin hormone. The ghrelin hormone is a hormone that is responsible for hunger. Low levels of ghrelin reduce the feeling of hunger even when you do not have any food in your system. As such, you can go for longer durations of time without eating (Brooks, 2018). In addition, an increase in the protein and vegetable intake also reduces appetite.

An increase in your level of focus and energy could also be a sign that your body has completely achieved the state of ketosis. Initially, when people start the ketogenic diet, there are usually many reports of brain-fog, sluggishness, and feeling sick. This has fondly been referred to as the 'keto flu.' This mainly occurs because the body is being made to change from using glucose as the primary source of energy to using ketone bodies. This is a major change and may require the body to undergo some changes which are responsible for the feeling of tiredness. As such, these symptoms are a good sign that your ketogenic diet is becoming effective.

However, in the long term, people experience improved memory and an increase in the levels of energy in the body. This is because ketone bodies are an extremely powerful source of energy for the brain.

Other common symptoms of ketosis include constipation, diarrhea, and a decrease in your exercise performance. These are however caused by the dietary shift and are therefore transitory in nature. Once the body gets used to the changes, your body functioning should be restored back to normal. Some of the temporary symptoms that are caused by dehydration and low carbohydrate levels are headaches, nausea, stomach pain, and lethargy.

To reduce or even eliminate some of the side effects of the ketogenic diet, you are advised to drink lots of water and other non-caloric drinks such as coffee to reduce the effects of dehydration. In addition, boost your intake of exogenous ketones which will reduce the time it will take for your body to enter the state of ketosis. This involves taking supplements and foods that are rich in ketone bodies. You could also increase your intake of fats as it will help you ease into the state of ketosis.

In addition, as you begin the ketogenic diet, make sure to prepare yourself mentally for some of these symptoms. This will be very important in keeping you motivated. Keep in mind that the ketogenic diet involves major changes to your body and you will need to give yourself time to fully adjust to the changes. Maintain a positive mindset and always bear in mind that the journey only gets better.

A List of People Who Should Not Use the Ketogenic Diet

Based on the extreme nature of the ketogenic diet, it is not suitable for everyone. Because of the inherent differences from one individual to the next, you may find that the keto diet may not work for everyone. Some people may experience crippling symptoms of the keto flu or severe PMS symptoms among other conditions. As such, before you begin your keto journey, you are advised to consult with your doctor so as to receive a go-ahead.

When you begin the dieting process, you will need to carefully monitor your body for any signs of weakness, dizziness, light-headedness, moodiness, or even constipation. While some of these signs and symptoms are perfectly normal when you begin the ketogenic diet, they are expected to disappear a few days into the diet. If you observe any severe symptoms, you are advised to stop the diet and consult the experts on the way forward. The suffering and discomfort that you will experience are simply not worth it.

Pregnant and lactating women are strongly advised against the ketogenic diet. This is because they have additional energy needs for the growing fetus and in the case of lactating women, for the growing baby who depends on breast milk for nourishment. Such women are advised to try out the diet once they have given birth and have breastfed for at least 6 months. Failure to do so, these women may find themselves risking the lives of both the babies and themselves as they may be severely malnourished in the process. Worse still, such women may develop even more complications.

If you are chronically stressed, then it probably is not a good idea for you to create additional stress for your body. The elevated heart rate, high blood pressure, and high levels of stress hormones from chronic stress are already taking a toll on your body. The ketogenic diet is only going to make your body more stressed, and you may not achieve your intended goals. This is because the low-carb diet causes a significant drop in the glucose levels in the bloodstream. This stimulates the body to release large amounts of the cortisol hormone, a stress hormone that increases the amount of glucose in the blood by breaking down glycogen and proteins.

While people who have both type 1 and type 2 diabetes could benefit from the ketogenic diet, they are strongly advised to first consult their medical practitioner before going forward. In some situations, the ketogenic has led to an increase in blood pressure and the cholesterol levels in the bod while in other situations, it has reduced the insulin levels and the blood pressure levels. As such, if you are interested in the ketogenic diet, you are advised to first seek the advice of your doctor.

Anyone who does not get the recommended eight hours of sleep is highly advised to avoid the ketogenic diet. This applies to all students who have to sleep late while studying or even people who are forced to work for long shifts. Inadequate sleep already stresses the body and affects your health. Dieting is likely to make your body deteriorate further. As such, you are more likely to experience feelings of weakness and lightheadedness.

People who have a history of eating disorders are also strongly advised against trying out the ketogenic diet. This is because such people already have a history of abnormal and disturbed eating habits, which include anorexia and bulimia nervosa. The diet may create additional problems for you which may make your situation worse than it already was.

If your lifestyle does not fit into the keto diet process, you should avoid forcing yourself to adopt it. This is because essentially, the ketogenic diet is meant to fit into your lifestyle and not the other way round. Forcing the diet may cause it to fail even before ketosis fully kicks in. You must, therefore, learn to respect your body and the signals it gives you.

Lastly, you should not get on the diet if you are not interested and most of all passionate about it. Being an extremely demanding process, you will only set yourself up for failure and miserableness, even before you get started. In addition, you should not adopt the diet if you are not armed with the necessary knowledge about everything to do with the diet. Again, you will only set yourself up for failure as knowledge is indeed   power.

Chapter 2: Benefits of the Ketogenic Diet

General Benefits of Keto

The ketogenic diet has widely grown in popularity because of the wide range of benefits that the diet offers. Unlike other low-carb diets, the ketogenic diet is a healthy and nutritious diet that is likely to improve your health and general well-being.

The main benefit that is associated with the ketogenic diet is weight loss. The diet gradually eases the body into a state of ketosis which is characterized by increased fat burning to provide the body with the energy that is required for normal functioning. During ketosis, the body burns down both the fats in the food as well as the body's fat reserves to generate energy.

As a result of the fat-burning mechanism, the ketogenic diet results in protection from obesity, cardiovascular disease, diabetes, and hypertension (high blood pressure). During the ketogenic diet, the insulin levels in the blood drop significantly, facilitating fat burning. The drop in insulin consequently leads to a drop in blood sugar levels, which decreases the risk of type 2 diabetes (Gunnars, 2016). A drop in insulin levels also leads to an increase in the breakdown of body fat, facilitating the use of fat as an energy source. This greatly reduces the cholesterol levels in the body and cases of obesity and cardiovascular diseases (Gunnars, 2016).

It results in an improvement in insulin sensitivity. As a result of the decreased insulin levels in the bloodstream, the body cells become more sensitive to any insulin released into the bloodstream. As such, it does not accumulate within the blood. Diabetes patients who consistently follow the ketogenic diet could find their doctors reducing or even completely removing their diabetes medication because of this.

In addition, during ketosis, there are elevated levels of ketones in the body which suppress the production of the ghrelin hormone. The ghrelin hormone is a hormone that is responsible for hunger. Low levels of ghrelin reduce your appetite and the feeling of hunger, even when you do not have any food in your system. As such, you can go for longer durations of time without eating. This ensures that you will pay more attention to the true hunger signals as opposed to cravings, reducing your daily caloric intake.

Retarded growth of tumors. The ketogenic diet leads to a decrease in the growth of cancerous tumors and increased sensitivity to chemotherapy. When cancerous cells are exposed to environments that contain lower glucose levels, proliferation, and cell death quickly follow. This is a process known as cell starvation. Today, there are some cancer patients who have been treated with the ketogenic diet mainly as a supplement to chemotherapy and in some situations, as the main treatment.

As we saw in the first chapter, the ketogenic diet was initially used as a dietary treatment for epileptic patients, specifically children. While most epileptic patients use anti-epileptic drugs (AED) to control seizures today, any patients who are unable to control their seizures are advised to use the ketogenic diet to control these symptoms. However, the diet should always be carried out with care and with the consent of a specialized medical practitioner. Thus far, the ketogenic diet has been famed for reducing seizures in epileptic children.

There is already strong scientific research that suggests that ketone bodies are a much more powerful source of fuel for the brain as compared to glucose. In addition, while a high intake of carbohydrates has been proven to damage the brain, ketone bodies have been proven to improve mental acuity. With this in mind, it has scientifically been proven that the ketogenic diet has the ability to reduce the progression of the Alzheimer's disease and even to reverse some of the effects.

One study involving the ketogenic diet that was conducted on animals suggested that the ketone molecules produced by the liver are important in protecting the brain from injuries and in aiding the brain to recover after a brain injury.

It reduces inflammation. Inflammation is a common symptom of all chronic diseases that we face today. It is known to occur whenever the body is trying to heal itself. However, whenever inflammation occurs for too long, it is associated with some negative effects.

A ketogenic diet involves increased consumption of foods that are rich in fats and oils. These high fats and oils decrease the production of Leukotriene B4 (LTB4) which is involved in various cellular processes that are related to inflammation (Delauer, 2018). Reduced inflammation will result in reduced pain and less digestive problems.

Preliminary research also seems to suggest that the ketogenic diet has a myriad of benefits to a variety of other diseases such as Parkinson's, fatty-liver disease, and migraines.

Women-specific Benefits

Did you know that eating healthy fats actually boosts fertility in women? This is because fats are involved in the creation of all your hormones. Eating the right type of foods, such as those that you enjoy on a ketogenic diet will ensure that your body produces all the required hormones to keep you healthy.

Estrogen and progesterone are integral in the normal

functioning of the female body. Whenever these two hormones are balanced to their normal levels, you will experience decreased menstrual cramps and less moodiness. This, in turn, will boost your fertility and even lead to better sex!

The hormonal balance that is caused by the healthy fats in the ketogenic diet results in additional benefits, which are even more pronounced in women. They include sound sleep, increased energy and drive, and improved libido.

Menopausal women are especially advised to get on the ketogenic diet. This is because sticking to the ketogenic diet will help to reduce some of the symptoms of menopause. The menopausal period is characterized by hot flushes especially at night, night sweats, irritability, high blood pressure, high cholesterol, insulin resistance, and slower metabolism among other symptoms.

Insulin control that comes with the ketogenic diet is believed to restore hormonal balance to menopausal women, reducing some of the common symptoms of menopause. Previous research done on women with the polycystic ovarian syndrome (PCOS) suggests that sex hormones are intricately linked to the insulin levels in the body. Hence, by improving your insulin levels through a high-fat and low-carb diet, you could balance out your sex hormones and reduce some of the symptoms of menopause such as weight gain, reduced metabolism, and reduced sex drive.

A ketogenic diet is also important to menopausal women as it facilitates weight loss. This is because weight gain is one of the common symptoms of menopause. More often than not, women will report increased weight around the abdominal area even when they are doing everything right. The primary cause of this weight loss is usually a decrease in the levels of estrogen which results in weight gain. A ketogenic diet helps menopausal women with weight management by increasing the rate at which fat is being burnt and boosting the body's metabolism. In addition, the moderate protein diet and the decreased production of the ghrelin hormone boost satiety, reducing the occurrence of cravings and hunger pangs which often result in weight gain.

Hot flushes and night sweats are some of the most annoying symptoms of menopause. Night sweats make you simultaneously feel hot and cold. They disrupt sleep and create a general feeling of discomfort. While the exact cause of hot flushes is still unknown, it is believed that they are caused by low levels of the estrogen hormone. Menopausal women on the ketogenic diet will, however, experience hormonal balance, reducing the occurrence of this symptom. In addition, the ketone bodies released during ketosis will reduce inflammation in the body which may improve the body's ability to regulate its temperatures.

A decrease in libido is one of the common symptoms of menopause which are caused by the fluctuation in the sex hormones. A ketogenic diet can, however, help with this as it will lead to the hormonal balance of both estrogen and progesterone, increasing your libido. In addition, a high-fat diet boosts the production of sex hormones which is important in maintaining a high level of libido.

Once the body fully shifts form the use of glucose to the use of ketones to fuel its organs, there is a decrease in the mood swings and energy dips that are caused by a high-carbohydrate diet. This is because the body now has an endless supply of ketone bodies, which are a more potent source of energy for the body as compared to glucose. Menopausal women are highly advised to get on this diet as it is likely to improve their energy levels.

Menopausal women are also prone to mood swings and irritation. Hormonal imbalance of estrogen and progesterone makes menopausal women very difficult to be around. This may negatively impact their personal and social lives, creating even more issues. However, through the ketogenic diet, hormonal balance is restored to the body and women are able to resume their happy and 'normal' state.

Chapter 3: The Ketogenic Diet for Women

Why is the Ketogenic Diet Different for Men and Women?

Your overall health and well-being is a three-part process that involves your diet, physical activity levels, and mindset. Before choosing a diet to follow, it is important for you to seek the advice of a medical practitioner or a nutritionist to get a go-ahead. In addition, it is important for you to research as much as possible so that you know everything there is to know about the diet.

The ketogenic diet is arguably one of the best dietary methods out there. As such, many people, both men and women get attracted to it thanks to the plethora of benefits that it has to offer. However, more often than not, women get discouraged from following this diet. This is because some health experts strongly advise women against this diet claiming that it negatively impacts a woman's hormones.

While it is true that the ketogenic diet affects the hormones of men and women alike, it is a myth that it negatively impacts the health of women. As a matter of fact, the only difference between men and women on the ketogenic diet is that the signs are more outward in women as compared to men. However, since women often rely on information on the internet and word-of-mouth to make their decisions, this misinformation greatly discourages women from trying out the ketogenic diet, even in situations where women would greatly benefit from it.

The truth of the matter is that the ketogenic diet is just different but not necessarily harmful to women. This is because the female body is biologically different from the male body. As such, a minor fluctuation in the nutrients consumed by a woman could have profound effects on the balance of the female sex hormones. In addition, the balance of sex hormones is closely linked to the overall health of a woman. Any imbalance is bound to pose a health challenge to the woman.

Women who experience irregular menstrual periods or gain weight while on the ketogenic diet must understand that these changes do not occur because of the state of ketosis. Missed or irregular periods are more often than not caused by weight loss more than they are caused by the ketogenic diet. The main effect of ketosis is usually weight loss. Sudden weight loss is usually associated with a sharp drop in estrogen which in turn leads to missed periods.

Due to the fear of consuming too much fat, women often consume very little fat while on the ketogenic diet. Since most of the fat is usually converted into ketone bodies by the liver, very little fat is left behind to create the vital sex hormones which are responsible for the menstrual cycle. This in turn negatively affects the menstrual cycle.

Failure to achieve the state of ketosis by consuming more than 5% of carbohydrates could also have a negative impact on the health of a woman. This is because carbohydrates are often associated with mood swings and irritability. In addition, when carbohydrates are broken down into glucose, any excess is stored in the form of fats. Hence, exceeding your specified daily carbohydrates intake has the potential of disrupting your hormonal distribution and could lead to weight loss.

Why do Women Struggle on the Ketogenic Diet?

Low-carb diets such as the ketogenic diet have been proven to elevate the levels of cortisol in the body. Cortisol is a stress hormone that is released by the body whenever the sugar levels in the bloodstream are low. By limiting the intake of carbohydrates to the extent that you do on the ketogenic diet, the body is triggered to enter the starvation mode. It is at this point that the cortisol hormone is released in order to increase the energy levels despite the low sugar levels. Being a glucocorticoid hormone, cortisol stimulates the gluconeogenesis process which allows the body to break down fats and proteins into sugar. In addition, cortisol and other stress hormones increase the body's insulin resistance.

This makes the ketogenic diet very stressful within the first few days. During this time, the cortisol levels in the bloodstream are usually elevated. As cortisol is a stress hormone, it will make you feel weak, fatigued, and stressed out. However, if you follow the ketogenic diet consistently, your body will shift to the state of ketosis within 3 – 4 days. This implies that your body will stop breaking down proteins for energy and will instead use fat as the primary source of fuel. The cortisol levels in the bloodstream will then decrease significantly as you will no longer need the hormone to increase the blood sugar levels.

Whenever the cortisol levels are elevated, the hormones in the body are completely destabilized, causing them to fluctuate significantly as a result of the elevated cortisol levels. Unlike men, women are sensitive to the slightest fluctuations in sex hormones. As such, the elevated stress levels are likely to cause irregular menstrual periods, decreased libido, infertility, raging PMS, premature menopause, unexplained weight gain, and a low mood and appetite.

Women must, however, realize that the elevated cortisol levels only occur when you begin the ketogenic diet and gradually decrease as you fully ease into the state of ketosis. As such, some of the above mentioned symptoms should disappear within the first few days. In the event that the symptoms persist, it is likely that external stressors are the problem.

Many women have been made to believe that the ketogenic diet has a negative effect on the thyroid gland and could lead to diseases and disorders such as hypothyroidism. The truth is that any negative criticism of the ketogenic diet based on the thyroid gland is simply false. Contrary to popular opinion, the diet actually has a positive impact on the normal thyroid functioning.

Medical practitioners unanimously agree that when it comes to healing the immune system, there is no better healer than the ketone molecules found in the bloodstream. These ketone bodies re-regulate the entire immune system, re-balancing the hormones in the process. Evidence seems to suggest that the ketogenic diet results in a decrease in a hormone known as T3 which is the most active thyroid hormone.

Most of the T3 hormone binds itself to protein, and the rest floats within the bloodstream. The hormone regulates the body's metabolism, temperature, and heart rate.

Many critics discredit the ketogenic diet by stating that a decrease in the T3 hormone could lead to hypothyroidism. However, just because the level of T3 is low does not mean that the thyroid will not function as it should. This is because hypothyroidism is mainly caused by elevated levels of the thyroid stimulating hormone (TSH) and low levels of T4 in the bloodstream. Reduced levels of T3 are normal and do not have any negative effect on the thyroid.

The main cause of the decrease in T3 while on the ketogenic diet is that the body is able to work more efficiently during ketosis. Scientists believe that the decrease in T3 could actually increase your life span. This is because the T3 cells make your body consume much more energy. This leads to a longer life span because it conserves energy and reduces free radical production. In addition, reduced levels of T3 are good for you as they allow you to lose weight without losing your muscle mass.

However, this is not to say that women should avoid the ketogenic diet. On the contrary, women are encouraged to adopt the ketogenic diet as it has been scientifically proven to be good for the female body. In addition, women who plan on starting the ketogenic diet are advised to consult with their doctors so as to come up with ways to manage the symptoms of the keto flu and any other side effects that may occur at the beginning of the diet.

Chapter 4: Building Blocks for the Perfect Ketogenic Diet

What Type of Foods should be considered for the Ketogenic Diet?

As we have mentioned before, there are about 4 types of ketogenic diets that are widely accepted around the globe. The Standard Ketogenic Diet (SKD) is by far the most popular type. It consists of 70% fats, 25% protein, and 5% carbohydrates.

The ketogenic diet, like many other dietary plans, involves the consumption of healthy and nutritious foods. The diet pays particular attention to both the quality and quantity of the foods that you consume to ensure that you achieve your desired goals. As such, foods that are considered for the ketogenic diet should contain all the important macro and micronutrients to contribute to good health and the general well-being of the person.

In addition, while starvation is essentially the deprivation of food and important nutrients, the ketogenic diet is simply a dietary plan that limits the amount of carbohydrates consumed so that the body can ease into the state of ketosis. As such, the foods consumed during the feeding window should be highly nutritious or else many other complications will come up, and the ketogenic diet may not work.

Nutrients are also important in ensuring that the biological process of autophagy is operational. Autophagy refers to the process by which the cells in the body can remove any junk in the bloodstream and recycle wastes. Malnourishment causes the autophagy process to slow down and may cause the cells to cannibalize and result in fast aging.

Nutritious meals are those that contain all the important macro and micronutrients that are required for the proper functioning of the body. Each meal should have a healthy portion of these nutritious recipes, implying that the meal should not be too big, nor too small.

Nutritious recipes are often rich in fruits and vegetables. It is highly recommended that each recipe should contain at least three different types of fruits and three different types of vegetables. This is because fruits and vegetables are very rich in both soluble and insoluble fibers.

Foods that are high in fiber are highly recommended for the ketogenic diet. The fiber contained in foods is broadly classified as either soluble or insoluble. However, both serve the functions of contributing to satiety, regulating the speed of digestion, and by extension, the rate at which glucose is absorbed into the bloodstream, reducing constipation and the risk of colon cancer. Fiber rich vegetables include broccoli, cucumbers, carrots, sprouts, beet roots, spinach, kale, and celery roots, among others.

First, foods that are rich in fiber are important in preventing constipation. This is because soluble fibers absorb a lot of water, making your stool softer and larger while insoluble fibers make your stool more bulky. As such, the stool is easily able to pass through your gut, preventing the constipated feeling.

Second, foods that are rich in fiber absorb a lot of water in the gut. They are then converted into a gel which makes the process of digestion take a longer time. This, in turn, has the effect of making you feel satiated for longer periods of time. Satiation then reduces the occurrence of any hunger pangs and cravings.

Foods that are rich in proteins are also highly recommended. Some of the benefits of proteins include reducing your appetite, cravings and hunger levels, boosting your metabolism and fat burning, contributing to increased muscles, and they are generally good for your bones. The proteins that you consume should be low carb, and the meats should be lean. This is because fatty cuts of beef or pork usually contain saturated fats, which are essentially unhealthy and could lead to increased cholesterol levels.

Fruits and vegetables are also of particular importance. Vegetables are known to contain fibers which take a long time to be digested in the gut. As such, these vegetables create a filling of satiation, keeping hunger pangs and cravings at bay. Fruits, on the other hand, are rich in minerals and vitamins, which boost your general body immunity and contribute to your wellbeing.

People are advised to avoid foods that are rich in saturated fats, refined sugars, and simple carbohydrates. These include red meats, white foods, and all foods that are prepared through deep-frying.

Fats and Oils

Fats make up at least 70% of your total daily caloric intake. This is because of the state of ketosis - from where the diet derives its name from – depends on fats stored in the adipose tissues as well as the dietary fats. During ketosis, the liver usually breaks down these fats to produce ketone bodies which act as an alternative source of fuel for the body.

As the bulk of the diet consists of fats, you are strongly advised to consume plenty of fats and oils from varied sources. Many people, especially women, have the tendency of consuming less fats and oils in the fear that they will gain weight as opposed to losing it. Since most of the fat is usually converted into ketone bodies by the liver, very little fat is left behind to create the vital sex hormones. This is considered a huge mistake, and it is one of the reasons why people fail to achieve their goals while on the ketogenic diet. It often leads to irregular menstrual periods and irritability in women.

While you are advised to maximize the intake of fats, you are also cautioned to stick to the smart fats. Smart fats are mono-saturated and saturated fats which are considered to be healthy for the body. They include ghee, grass-fed butter, coconut oil, macadamia oil, bone marrow, chicken fat, duck fat, egg yolk, sea food, fish oil, lard, and MCT oil.

Medium-chain triglycerides (MCTs) are keto-friendly as they are rapidly taken up by the liver and converted into ketones for energy. This results in an increase in the ketone bodies in the blood, increasing your overall energy levels. MCTs are contained in coconut oil, making it one of the best oils for the ketogenic diet. It has been shown to increase the body's metabolic rate, making it easier to lose weight, especially around the belly area.

Sea fish and shell fish are typically very keto-friendly as they contain numerous minerals and nutrients and are either free of carbohydrates or low in carbohydrates. While the amounts of carbohydrates in different shellfish vary, shrimp and most types of crabs are known to contain no carbohydrates. In addition, some sea fish such as salmon, sardines, and mackerels are known to contain high amounts of omega-3 oils which are essential in lowering insulin levels and increasing insulin sensitivity especially in overweight and obese people.

Avocados are considered to be extremely healthy. They are high in various minerals and nutrients and low in carbohydrates, making them perfect for the ketogenic diet. They are high in potassium, an important mineral which makes the transition into ketosis smoother and easier for the body.

Similarly, eggs are also considered to be some of the healthiest foods on the planet. It is scientifically proven that one egg contains about 1 gram of carbohydrates and 6 grams of proteins, making it perfect for the ketogenic diet which is essentially low-carb and moderate-protein in nature. Eggs are believed to reduced hunger pangs and food cravings. The yolk is especially rich in nutrients and is important for the health of some vital body organs such as the heart and the eye.

Unhealthy fats should be avoided at all costs as they could result in elevated cholesterol levels and heart disease. You should avoid hydrogenated fats, trans fats, polyunsaturated fats, and other processed vegetable oils. This implies that you should avoid sunflower, soybean, canola, corn, cotton seed, and grapeseed oils at all costs.

Protein

Foods that are rich in proteins are also known as body-building foods mainly because they contain important amino acids which form the building blocks of our muscles and cellular structure. Proteins are either derived from animal or plant products, with many nutritionists highly recommending plant to animal protein.

Proteins should make up at least 25% of your total daily caloric intake.

Vegetables

Vegetables are some of the important foods that you will need during the ketogenic diet. This is because they contain plenty of nutrients, including but not limited to vitamin C, vitamin A, vitamin D, sodium, magnesium, potassium, and folic acid. Potassium may lower your blood pressure, decrease the chances of developing kidney stones, and reduce your bone loss (Biswas, 2018). Vegetables are also known to reduce the risk of heart disease and the chances of developing cancer.

In as much as vegetables are known to be rich in nutrients and vitamins, they are also a sneaky source of carbohydrates, which could be detrimental to the ketogenic diet. Your ketogenic diet food lists should, therefore, consist of vegetables that are low in carbohydrates but rich in nutrients.

Root vegetables are rich in carbohydrates. In some situations, they are also known as starchy vegetables due to their high starch content. You should make a point to limit your intake of moderately starchy foods and completely avoid vegetables that are rich in starch. Moderately starchy vegetables include leeks, beetroots, carrots, sweet potatoes, and parsnips. All other types of potatoes should be avoided at all costs as they are extremely high in starch.

The general rule of thumb is that the leafy and cruciferous vegetables are the best for the ketogenic diet. Not only are they low in carbohydrates, but they have also been linked to a decrease in the risk of developing cancer and heart disease. During preparation, these vegetables should always be lightly cooked. The vegetables include kales, broccoli, and cauliflower. They are often used as a substitute for the foods that are rich in carbohydrates.

Preparing a Meal Plan

The ketogenic diet has everything to do with calorie restriction, however, do not be fooled, food quality is just as important as food quantity. Successful weight loss using the ketogenic diet necessitates the use of a three-step approach that consists of a positive mindset, physical activity exercises, and healthy and nutritious recipes. Healthy recipes ensure that although the calorie intake is greatly restricted, the body and its vital organs receive all the important macro and micronutrients.

There are many foods that you could choose from to make a delicious meal that is still in line with the ketogenic diet. Below are some of the foods that constitute a healthy recipe:

Vegetables such as turnips, cauliflower, tomatoes, beetroot, broccoli, scallions, lettuce, bell peppers, spinach, cucumber, and kales. These vegetables are best eaten raw or lightly steamed or boiled to avoid destroying important nutrients and vitamins.

Fruits such as bananas, pineapples, grapes, strawberries, blueberries, lemon, lime, oranges, apples, tangerines, peaches, plums, gooseberries, and acai berries are also very important.

Nuts and seeds such as almonds, walnuts, pistachios, pecan, macadamia, sunflower seeds, pumpkin seeds, and melon seeds.

Proteins from foods such as chicken breast, lean cuts of pork and beef, tofu, eggs, beans, peas, black peas, and chickpeas. Many scientists recommend the use of plant-based protein as opposed to animal-based protein since it is widely believed that plant-based proteins are healthier and lead to longevity.

Whole grains from foods such as brown rice, oat, millet, quinoa, barley, and sorghum. These are cereals that are hardly refined and are considered to be healthy.

Healthy fats and oils from foods such as olive oil, peanut butter, coconut oil, almond butter, avocadoes, and sunflower butter.

Healthy calorie-free beverages such as unsweetened teas, coffees, homemade lemonade, coconut water, freshly made fruit juices, and most importantly, mineral water.

Once you begin your ketogenic diet, you should always schedule time to plan your meals. This, of course, involves creating time to visit the local market to stock up your kitchen cabinets and refrigerator. This section will provide you with guidance on some of the foods that you could include in your meal plan and those that are strictly forbidden. Hence, this will give you some guidance to help you with meal planning. As a disclaimer, you must note that the foods are not limited to those listed in this section.

Once you begin your ketogenic diet, you could choose a recipe from the above list of recipes. The recipes for the ketogenic diet are widely available across the internet and print media. As such, do not feel limited to the ones that we have listed in this section. You can always try out different recipes and stick to specific ones, depending on the recipes that you like best.

In addition, you must always remember to purchase what you can afford. Do not try to break the bank as you try to recreate some of the recipes that are listed here or those that you may have read from other sources. Always remember that the ketogenic diet is meant to fit into your lifestyle and not the other way round. Besides, a little creativity in the kitchen will go a long way.

Chapter 5: Hormones and Nutrition

Hormones in Women

This far, we can agree that the ketogenic diet does affect women more than it does men. However, this is not a reason to dismiss the diet as it offers a plethora of benefits which are important for the overall health and nutrition of the human body. We have seen that the ketogenic diet does indeed affect the hormones in women. However, this is not to say that the diet affects the hormones negatively. As a matter of fact, the ketogenic diet does have proven benefits for females suffering from endometriosis and uterine fibroids among many other conditions.

The ketogenic diet is considered to be tricky for women. This is not to say that it is impossible. The complications in women arise because the female body is extremely sensitive to changes in nutrients. In addition, hormonal balance, specifically the balance of sex hormones, is closely tied to a woman's overall health and nutrition. Any disruption in health and nutrition is likely to have a ripple effect on the health of a woman, further leading to some health conditions.

In order to understand how it is that the balance of sex hormones affects the health of a female, you will first need to understand the delicate role that sex hormones play in the female body. Hence, in this chapter, we analyze the role of female sex hormones.

The Role of Female Sex Hormones

Hormones are chemical messengers in the body which are produced by the endocrine glands. In essence, they control and co-ordinate different bodily functions. The endocrine system usually releases these hormones into the bloodstream after which they are transported to specific cells and tissues where the hormones will have an effect. They control most if not all of the major bodily functions. Some of the bodily functions that are controlled by the hormones include the feeling of hunger, growth, reproduction, emotion, metabolism, the use of energy, and even response to danger and stress, among many other functions.

Female sex hormones, also known as sex steroids, are the main hormones which are produced in the ovaries. The female sex hormones are estrogen, testosterone, and progesterone. Estrogen is considered to be the main sex hormone for women as it is responsible for many of the bodily changes that women experience during and after puberty all the way to menopause.

Estrogen and progesterone have been scientifically proven to have an effect on sleep patterns, mood, and mental functioning. The hormones, like all other hormones, act everywhere in the body, including in the brain. As such, they are believed to affect the levels of neurotransmitters that are released into the bloodstream. Estrogen, for example, is believed to increase the production of serotonin as well as the number of serotonin receptors in the brain. Serotonin is popularly known as a happy chemical as it contributes to the general happiness and wellbeing of an individual. Elevated levels of estrogen are therefore associated with feelings of happiness and joy while low levels of estrogen are known to lead to depression, panic attacks, and mood swings which are common symptoms in menopausal and pre-menopausal women.

Estrogen plays a crucial role in the growth, maturity, and metabolism of bone structures in both males and females at different ages. The hormone usually supports the intestinal absorption of calcium back into the bloodstream as well as the body's general retention of calcium. Calcium is considered to be one of the most important minerals to the human body as it contributes to the strength of the teeth and bones. As such, once it is absorbed, the mineral is usually transported to the bones, aiding in the proper growth and development of bone structures. Low estrogen levels reduce the body's ability to retain and consume calcium, leading to bone loss and a decrease in bone density. This explains why it is that pre-menopausal and menopausal women are at high risk of developing osteoporosis.

The progesterone hormone is intricately linked to the thyroid gland and consequently to the production of the thyroid hormones. The thyroid gland is the largest of the endocrine glands and is responsible for the regulation of body temperature and the rate of metabolism of different organs. This greatly affects the way in which all the bodily organs operate as it determines the energy levels available for different body functions. Progesterone is in turn responsible for stimulating the production of TPO and improving the signaling mechanism of the thyroid gland. TPO is an enzyme that is responsible for the production of thyroid hormones. Low levels of progesterone suppress the production of TPO, reducing the production of thyroid hormones. Low production of thyroid hormones leads to hot flushes and feelings of fatigue which are symptoms of hypothyroidism.

As we have mentioned before, like all other hormones, estrogen produced in the ovaries is released into the bloodstream and transported to specific body parts where it will have an effect. However, unlike other hormones, estrogen is believed to have an effect on virtually all organs and systems. As such, estrogen is also responsible for cardiovascular health in women.

Estrogen stimulates an increase in the production of HDL cholesterol, which is considered to be good for the body and a decrease in the production of LDL which is the harmful type of cholesterol. The hormone also promotes the relaxation and dilation of blood vessels which promotes the flow of blood in the body. It also enhances the blood clot formation process. A drop in the estrogen levels in the bloodstream leads to an increase in HDL cholesterol, which leads to a buildup of fat in the blood vessels, increasing the risk of a heart attack or even stroke, which are common symptoms in menopausal women.

The progesterone hormone leads to increased susceptibility of the human body to diseases and infections, lowering the body's immunity. In as much as this is considered to be a bad thing, it could also be a good thing as it often leads to the suppression of inflammation. Inflammation is one of the main immunity responses to diseases and infections in the body. Suppressing inflammation is often a good thing in the case of chronic diseases since inflammation only serves to make the symptoms worse.

There are many more functions of the female sex hormones in the body. However, these are the main functions of the hormones in relation to the ketogenic diet. Next, we will analyze some of the effects of hormonal imbalance caused by the ketogenic diet.

Insulin and Hormonal Imbalance

Besides the female sex hormones listed above, insulin is another major hormone that contributes to hormonal imbalance in women. Unlike the ketogenic diet, many diets made for women are usually high in refined sugars and low in healthy fats. Many of these foods are usually labeled as healthy or low fat, attracting many women to consume them. The consumption of these foods usually leads to a rapid increase in blood sugar levels, which as we mentioned before usually has a myriad of side effects. To compensate for the rise in glucose levels, the body increases its production of insulin, leading to a sharp decrease in blood sugar levels. The decrease is however usually short-lived as most of the body organs cannot survive without a steady supply of energy.

Due to the elevated stress levels caused by a decrease in the blood sugar levels, the body produces the cortisol hormone. The hormone is responsible for increasing the blood sugar levels by either breaking down the fat reserves to produce glucose or breaking down proteins to produce more glucose to provide energy to the body organs. The rise in blood sugar levels is consequently accompanied by a rise in insulin levels. The glucose is then transported within the bloodstream to specific cells and organs either for energy or for storage. This process, however, results in more craving for refined and processed foods.

However, over time, the cells lose their ability to absorb glucose, resulting in a condition known as insulin resistance. At this point, the insulin receptors in the cells usually alter their shape such that the insulin can no longer fit in the receptor. This implies that the insulin can no longer transport the glucose across the cell membrane. The insulin and glucose are both left to circulate within the bloodstream, resulting in high blood sugar levels.

When the cells are unable to absorb additional glucose, the body will convert the glucose in the bloodstream to fat. The accumulated fat cells will then serve as an endocrine organ, engaging in the production of additional estrogen. In addition, the elevated cortisol levels will lead to an increase in the conversion of progesterone to cortisol, leading to a decrease in the progesterone levels in the bloodstream.

Elevated levels of estrogen and reduced levels of progesterone will often lead to estrogen dominance. Estrogen dominance is a form of hormonal imbalance that is characterized by PMS-like symptoms such as mood swings, irritability, depression, and fatigue, among others.

Effects of Hormonal Imbalance in Women

The ketogenic diet emphasizes on high amounts of fat, moderate amounts of protein, and low amounts of carbohydrates. This has the effect of reducing and destabilizing the intake of nutrients in the body. The change in nutrient intake has the effect of destabilizing hormone production in the body, leading to hormonal imbalance.

Hormonal imbalance is the malfunction of hormones in the body which can cause even more health complications. Essentially, hormonal changes take place throughout a person's life, all the way from birth to death. However, the imbalance that is experienced by women on the ketogenic diet is not natural and should be controlled. Some of the effects of hormonal imbalance in women include:

PMS (Premenstrual Syndrome), is one of the common symptoms of hormonal imbalance in women. Some of the symptoms of PMS include mood swings, irritability, depression, food cravings, and fatigue. These symptoms are linked to a decrease in the levels of serotonin. This is because the imbalance of estrogen, specifically the decrease in the production of estrogen, often leads to a decrease in the production of serotonin.

The imbalance of the main female sex hormones, estrogen and progesterone could lead to the buildup of the uterine lining or could prevent the uterine walls from lining all together. This is because estrogen is responsible for the thickening of the uterine walls while progesterone is responsible for the thinning and shedding off of the uterine walls. Any imbalance, such that there are higher levels of estrogen and lower levels of progesterone could lead to a buildup of the uterine lining, which could result in a heavier menstrual flow and possibly the growth of fibroids. Elevated levels of progesterone, on the other hand, could lead to missed periods.

Polycystic Ovary Syndrome, popularly shortened as PCOS is a condition that is often characterized by missed menstrual periods, unwanted hair growth, acne, and difficulties in getting pregnant. It is caused by hormonal imbalance such as that which occurs to women on the ketogenic diet. Whenever the levels of insulin or a hormone known as LH are too high, the ovaries are stimulated to produce high amounts of testosterone. Testosterone is essentially a male hormone which should be produced in small quantities in the case of women. Whenever the levels of testosterone are higher than they should, women will report the above-named symptoms.

The hormones estrogen, testosterone, and leptin have been scientifically proven to contribute to weight gain and obesity. This is because the hormones usually influence the distribution of fat. They also affect appetite and metabolism. Elevated levels of either estrogen or testosterone in women encourage the accumulation of body fat, especially around the stomach area, leading to obesity.

On the other hand, obesity is also considered to cause hormonal imbalance. People who are obese are considered to have too much fat stored in the body. This fat usually acts as an endocrine organ, and it produces the estrogen hormone. This leads to elevated levels of estrogen in the bloodstream which lead to PMS-like symptoms in women.

Dietary and Lifestyle Interventions to Treat

Hormonal Imbalance

Luckily, hormonal imbalance is a condition that can be treated using some of the key dietary principles embodied in the ketogenic diet. As a cautionary measure, once you are diagnosed with hormonal imbalance, it will be prudent for you to consult the advice of a nutritionist or medical practitioner to determine the feasibility of using the ketogenic diet to manage the condition. People with certain conditions such as diabetes may be discouraged from using the diet. In some cases, the medical practitioner could modify the ketogenic diet to suit your needs.

Below are some of the dietary and lifestyle measures that you could adopt to manage hormonal imbalance. They all are in line with the ketogenic diet!

Focus on consuming a healthy and balanced diet for all your meals. Your diet should be 70% fats, 25% protein, and 5% carbohydrates. Despite the low carbohydrate intake, you should still ensure that you get all the macro and micronutrients that your body needs. As we mentioned earlier, the consumption of nutrients is usually intricately linked to the overall health and hormonal balance in women. As such, this is especially important for women since a stable intake of nutrients will reduce the imbalance of hormones.

Your intake of carbohydrates should contain foods that have a low glycemic count to reduce the amount of glucose circulating in your system. As we have mentioned, foods that have a high glycemic count are easily broken down into glucose, resulting in insulin resistance and estrogen dominance. Avoid sweets and foods containing wheat and flour as they essentially have a high glycemic count. Focus on home-cooked cereals as opposed to the refined and processed cereals and vegetables and grains that contain less starch.

Increase your consumption of healthy fats and oils and reduce your consumption of unhealthy fats. Hydrogenated fats, trans fats, and saturated fats are considered to be unhealthy as they are usually difficult to break down and often lead to elevated cholesterol levels. This implies that you should avoid all vegetable, soy, safflower, corn, and canola oils. Instead, you should focus on healthier fats found in fish such as sardines, mackerel, herring, and salmon, flax seeds, olive oil, macadamia oil, avocado oil, and coconut oil.

You should avoid consuming large portions of food at any point in time even though the food may be healthy. Instead, focus on having about 3 – 4 small meals at regular intervals in the course of the day. Large meals will cause your blood sugar levels to spike, a situation which could result in extreme mood swings, irritability, and depression. In addition, the smaller meals will reduce your total calorie intake while maintaining your supply of all the required macro and micronutrients.

Avoid all sweetened drinks, artificial sweeteners, and foods with preservatives and colorings as they are essentially high in sugars such as fructose and could lead to hormonal imbalance. This implies that you should avoid all sodas, energy drinks, fruit juices, and high-fructose corn syrup.

You should also avoid all dairy and meat products. These products usually contain hormones such as estrogen, progesterone, and prolactin. While these foods are good for the ordinary person, they are not recommended for individuals with hormonal imbalance as they could worsen the imbalance of hormones in the system, making some of the effects of imbalance possibly worse.

Regular exercise is also very important in restoring your hormonal balance. Both exercise and dietary changes are complimentary, implying that one cannot work without the other. Exercise alters the body's metabolism and fat distribution. In addition, regular exercise also alters the shape of the insulin receptors, making them compatible with the insulin. This is important in the reduction of insulin resistance as the insulin will then be able to transport glucose across the cell membrane. A reduction in the glucose in the bloodstream will result in a reduction in fats. This implies that less estrogen will be released from the fat cells, reducing the occurrence of estrogen dominance.

It is also very important to increase your consumption of foods that are high in fiber. Besides reducing constipation, foods that are rich in dietary fiber are known to reduce the rate at which glucose is absorbed into the bloodstream. This will reduce any cravings for sugary foods, reducing the amount of carbohydrates that you will be taking. In addition, foods that are rich in fibers will reduce your general appetite by reducing the occurrence of hunger pangs. Decreased calorie intake will, in turn, result in stable blood sugar levels which are likely to stabilize the hormones in the body.

Chapter 6: Everything that you need to Know about Growing Older

Perimenopause

Menopause is a widely-known phase that occurs in older women, mostly those in their mid-40s and 50s. While the phase is popularly known, many people do not know that there are several stages within the entire process, each with distinct symptoms and characteristics. The two stages within menopause are known as perimenopause and pre-menopause.

The perimenopause stage is just one of the two stages, and it occurs before the menopausal stage. On the other hand, we also have the pre-menopause stage which just like perimenopause occurs before menopause. Women going through this stage will have no symptoms of going through either menopause or perimenopause. They will still experience their periods and will be considered to be reproductive. However, they will be experiencing some hormonal changes which will not have any noticeable effects on the body. Unlike the pre-menopause stage, women in the perimenopause stage will begin experiencing some symptoms of menopause. While many people use the two words interchangeably, it is important to note that there is a key difference between the two.

Perimenopause, as the word suggests, refers to the period around menopause. It is also widely referred to as the menopause transition or climacteric. It is a phase that usually takes place in women several years before menopause and which lasts for about 4 to 8 years. While the average length of this stage is 4 years, it may go up to 10 years in some women. However, it is important to note that some women do not experience perimenopause. Instead, they begin their menopause directly.

Generally, women begin to experience perimenopause at different ages, depending on a number of factors such as their smoking history, family genetics, and cancer treatment, among many other factors. Women typically begin to notice the signs of early progression towards menopause in their 40's. However, it is not uncommon for some women to experience these signs as early as their mid-30s.

The end of the perimenopause phase usually marks the end of a woman's reproductive life. The end of the phase is said to have occurred when a woman goes for a period of 12 months without receiving their period. As such, the end of the perimenopause phase marks the beginning of the menopausal phase in a woman's life.

As we have mentioned before, the ovaries are part of the endocrine system. Their main function is to produce the female sex hormones, estrogen, and progesterone. Thus, during perimenopause, the ovaries gradually adjust their production of estrogen and progesterone as the body prepares itself for menopause and the cessation of the menstrual cycle. The levels of estrogen and progesterone in the system are therefore likely to increase and decrease sporadically, leading to irregular periods, among other symptoms of perimenopause.

In the last year and in some cases the last two years before menopause, the ovaries will significantly reduce their production of estrogen. However, despite the low levels of estrogen, it is still possible to get pregnant. As the levels of estrogen decrease further, menopause will only kick in at the point where the estrogen levels are so low that the ovaries can no longer release any eggs. It is at this point that menstruation will actually stop.

Perimenopause is a completely normal and gradual process that takes place in all women. However, in some cases, women may enter the perimenopause stage earlier than usual due to some risk factors highlighted below.

Women who come from families that have a history of early menopause are at high risk of beginning their menopausal symptoms earlier than other women. In addition, women who are frequent and heavy smokers are also likely to begin their menopause early. Cigarette smoke is believed to contain chemicals and substances which alter the balance of endogenous hormones such as estrogen and progesterone, leading to early menopause. In addition, nicotine contained in cigarettes is believed to elevate the cortisol levels in the body.

Perimenopause could also be treatment induced. Hormonal therapy, chemotherapy, surgical removal of both ovaries, and radiation therapy to the pelvis is believed to cause menopause to begin earlier than expected. The effects of these treatments may either be permanent or temporary, depending on the age of the woman at the time of treatment. The effects are likely to be more permanent in women who are already several years into pre-menopause or perimenopause and more temporary in younger women. Other factors that determine the occurrence of treatment-induced menopause include the type of drug, the dosage, and the length of treatment. Treatment-induced menopause is usually diagnosed by a physical examination, questions on the symptoms experienced, and a blood test to determine the hormonal levels.

During perimenopause, you might experience some of the signs and symptoms listed below, some which may be subtle and unnoticeable and others which are not subtle. They are:

Irregular Periods: As the levels of estrogen and progesterone fluctuate irregularly, the process of ovulation, and consequently menstruation, becomes less predictable. You may find yourself skipping some periods altogether due to very low levels of estrogen in the bloodstream. Alternatively, the time between your periods may either be longer than usual or shorter than usual. Due to the presence of less progesterone to regulate the growth of the uterine lining, you may find that your period is either heavier than usual or lighter than usual. Some women may even experience the growth of fibroids or even endometriosis due to the low levels of estrogen.

Mood swings: Perimenopause-related hormonal changes are believed to result in depression, irritability, and anxiety. While we do not dismiss that the mood changes may be caused by other factors, it is believed that about 10%-20% of women experience mood changes during perimenopause. Other factors that are likely to cause mood changes include a history of depression, mid-life stress, and general poor health.

Sleeping Problems: Insomnia is believed to be a common symptom among both men and women as they age. However, scientists have established a strong causal relationship between the occurrence of night sweats and sleep disturbances. Many women experiencing perimenopause have reported that sleep becomes irregular and sometimes even unpredictable.

Changes in sexual drive: During perimenopause, many women experience a decrease in sexual desire. Sexual arousal becomes even more difficult, a factor which may frustrate your sexual partner. However, if you have been having satisfactory sexual intercourse before menopause, then it is highly likely that this will not change even after menopause.

Hot flushes and night sweats: Hot flushes and heavy sweating at night are common symptoms of perimenopause. As you grow older and approach menopause, these symptoms will most probably increase in intensity and duration. The sleep problems experienced by women in their perimenopause stage are to a large extent caused by the hot flushes and night sweats.

Vaginal and bladder issues: As the levels of estrogen decrease further, some women are likely to experience vaginal dryness and elasticity as the tissues in the vagina become less lubricated. This is believed to be the main reason for the painful sex that is experienced during perimenopause. Vaginal dryness may also cause itchiness and irritation. The loss of vaginal tissue due to the low levels of estrogen may cause urinary incontinence, characterized by the leakage of urine especially when one coughs or sneezes or persistent urine urgency. Women at this stage are also more susceptible to urinary-tract infections.

Decreased fertility: Due to the imbalance of the major sex hormones and the irregularity of the menstrual cycle, women are less likely to become pregnant. However, this is not to say that it is impossible to become pregnant. As long as you are experiencing your periods, however irregular, you could still get pregnant. If your goal is to conceive, then worry not, there are still some treatments that are available to ensure that you get pregnant and carry your baby to term.

Other common symptoms of perimenopause include fatigue, worse Premenstrual Syndrome (PMS), breast tenderness, difficulties in concentration, headaches, and fatigue.

Menopause

Menopause is a natural process that occurs in women immediately after the perimenopause stage. As women grow older, they consistently produce lower levels of the main female sex hormones, estrogen and progesterone. In response to the low hormone levels, the female body will undergo some major changes. One of the most common symptoms of the onset of menopause is the occurrence of irregular periods or missed periods all together. As such, menopause is said to have begun when a woman goes for a period of 12 months without receiving their menstrual period. These menopausal symptoms are said to begin anywhere from 40 years of age all the way to 50 years of age.

Although menopause is a naturally occurring biological process, it may be induced by some external factors. One of the main external factors that may cause the occurrence of menopause is the surgical removal of either one or both of the ovaries, also known as oophorectomy. As you probably know by now, the ovaries are part of the endocrine system as they are the main organs that produce the female sex hormones. The removal of the ovaries will result in a significant decrease in the levels of estrogen and progesterone circulating in the body, signaling the beginning of menopause.

Ovarian ablation could also induce the beginning of menopause. Ovarian ablation refers to the shutdown of the functions of the ovary. It is usually caused by surgery, hormone therapy, and radiotherapy in women with tumors. Pelvic radiation could also adversely affect the ovaries, which are located in the pelvic region. Lastly, any injuries to the pelvic region could also signal the beginning of some menopausal symptoms. These injuries may cause the damage or even the destruction of the ovaries, resulting in a decrease in the production of the major female sex hormones and consequently the occurrence of menopause. In such cases, the menopausal symptoms are likely to begin earlier than expected, depending on the severity.

The symptoms of menopause are much like the symptoms of perimenopause. The only difference is probably the degree or severity of the signs and symptoms. Nonetheless, we will still list the symptoms of menopause, making sure to add some of the symptoms that are specific to menopause. Below are the signs and symptoms of menopause:

Psychological Symptoms: These include the feelings of

anxiety, irritability, depression, lack of confidence, confusion, panic attacks, feelings of invisibility, and even mood swings. These symptoms may either be caused by the physical changes that occur during the rebalancing of the hormones or may directly be caused by the hormonal imbalance that occurs during menopause. However, the fluctuation of the levels of estrogen and progesterone is considered to be the main cause. These symptoms are considered to be the most problematic symptoms of menopause due to their unpredictable nature.

Sleep problems: Women experiencing menopause find it difficult to sleep because of the chills, night sweats, and hot flushes that occur as a result of hormonal imbalance. Hot flushes are said to occur when an individual experiences a sudden onset of feverish heat. Severe hot flushes are known as night sweats. These night sweats occur at night and could cause your bed sheets and clothes to get drenched in sweat. It is important to note that these night sweats and hot flushes could also occur during the day. In some situations, some women may experience chills as soon as the night sweats and hot flushes reduce.

Weight gain and slow metabolism: Many women will experience weight gain especially around the abdomen and stomach area. As a result, some women will find their body shape changing during menopause. This gain in weight is not usually caused by increased food intake but is instead caused by the hormonal changes that occur during menopause. Estrogen, in particular, is believed to be crucial in controlling body weight by regulating the rate of metabolism in our bodies. A slow metabolism can, therefore, be attributed to a decrease in the production of estrogen.

Hair problems: During menopause, most if not all women begin to experience some obvious changes in their hair. Suddenly, women will report reduced hair on the head and increased hair on other unwanted areas such as the face, hands, chest, neck, back, and the legs. This symptom is usually very confusing and embarrassing to most women. In addition, the hair in the head will become very thin and will grow much more slowly.

These changes mainly occur due to the decrease in the levels of estrogen and progesterone in the body. The female sex hormones are usually responsible for hair growth. Hence, when the levels decrease, as they do during menopause, the hair becomes thinner and grows much more slowly. In addition, the decrease in the female sex hormones usually stimulates the increased production of androgens, the male sex hormones. These hormones usually case the hair follicles to become smaller, resulting in thinner hair strands. The hormones may also cause the hair follicles to grow in unwanted regions, hence the growth of chin hair during menopause.

Reduced bone mass: Many women will report increased pain in their joints during menopause. In fact, many women in their late 40s and early 50s are diagnosed with osteoporosis, a disease that is characterized by the thinning of the bone mass. The hormonal changes that take place during menopause are believed to interfere with the natural process of building bones. This is because estrogen is usually responsible for the preservation of calcium in the body and the absorption of more calcium from the small intestines. A decrease in the production of estrogen will result in an increased bone breakdown, resulting in decreased bone mass and increased pain in the joints.

Vaginal and bladder issues: Vaginal dryness and elasticity is yet another common symptom of menopause. It mainly occurs due to the decreased lubrication of the vagina due to hormonal imbalance experienced during menopause. Vaginal dryness is then believed to cause itchiness and irritation in the vaginal area. In addition, during menopause, some women will experience the loss of vaginal tissue which is usually caused by a decrease in the production of estrogen in the body. The loss of vaginal tissue may result in urinary incontinence and urinary urgency. This implies that it gets difficult to hold in urine, especially when coughing or sneezing.

Loss of muscle mass: Due to the reduced rate of metabolism, some women will experience a decrease in muscle mass. The breasts will lose their fullness and the skin may begin to sag or to get wrinkles.

Other signs and symptoms of menopause include insomnia, reduced sex drive, a racing heartbeat, urinary tract infections, and sore breasts, among others. It is important to note that the symptoms of menopause vary from one individual to another depending on other factors such as genetics. Some women may experience all the symptoms of menopause while others may only experience one or two.

While some of the changes that occur during menopause are perfectly normal and part of the natural biological process, they may cause a lot of physical discomfort and could also affect your emotional health. As such, you should regularly visit your doctor for consultation on how to manage the symptoms as well as to get preventive health care.

Due to the increased discomfort caused by some of the symptoms of menopause, it is important to come up with different ways to manage these symptoms such that life becomes more comfortable. Generally, you could adopt some alternative treatments, lifestyle changes, and even home remedies to reduce some of these symptoms. Below are some of the tips to help you manage the symptoms of menopause:

Supplement your diet using vitamins and minerals such as magnesium, vitamin D, calcium, flax seeds, and soy to increase your bone mass and by extension, to reduce the chances of developing osteoporosis, to increase your energy levels, and to improve your sleeping patterns. It is, however, important to consult your doctor to advise you on the mineral supplements that you will need.

In addition, it is important to keep your body cool and comfortable at all times. This could be through dressing in loose clothing, especially at night to prevent the effects of the hot flushes and night sweats. In addition, you should keep your environment cool and airy by ensuring that there is proper ventilation. When sleeping, avoid heavy blankets to reduce the occurrence of night sweats. You could also install a fan in your bedroom to help with the night sweats or alternatively, purchase a portable fan to keep you cool at all times.

Come up with ways to exercise your body and to manage your weight. The ketogenic diet is one way that will ensure that you lose any extra pounds while you reap some benefits for your overall health. Exercising for about 20 – 30 minutes daily is also important to ensure that you do not gain any weight. Some of the other benefits of exercising include increased energy levels, improved moods, good sleep, and overall better health.

Women are also advised to reduce their calorie intake, a factor which is often responsible for the weight gain. This implies that you may need to cut your intake of sweet and sugary foods. While reducing your calorie intake, you must make sure that you do not compromise on your daily nutritional needs by consuming more fruits, vegetables, and whole grains as opposed to starches and highly-processed foods which are rich in calories.

In the event that you experience the psychological symptoms of menopause, you are advised to seek the services of a psychiatrist or therapist so as to deal with the feelings of depression, anxiety, irritability, and sadness that you may be feeling. Alternatively, you could speak to your friends and family about these symptoms.

Avoid the habit of smoking and limit your intake of alcohol. It has been scientifically proven that tobacco smoke contains chemicals and substance which affect the balance of hormones in the body. Continued smoking could, therefore, make the symptoms of menopause even worse by causing the hormonal levels to fluctuate even further. In addition, continued smoking and intake of alcohol could lead to further complications such as cancer, heart diseases, and lung damage. The same applies to the intake of alcohol.

Chapter 7: Conquering Stress

Cortisol Hormone

As you are aware by the now, the main principle behind the ketogenic diet is the fat-burning mechanism that occurs when the body goes into the state of ketosis. The keto diet is essentially high in fats, moderate in protein, and low in carbohydrates. Hence, some people may refer to it as a Very Low Carb Diet (VLCD).

When you consume food that contains carbohydrates, the enzymes in the digestive system will break it down into glucose. Glucose is the primary source of energy for the body organs and the cellular structures. Low glucose levels are usually experienced during situations of starvation and fasting. Hence, low glucose levels are not normal and in some situations, may even be harmful to your health.

When you first begin the keto diet, the levels of glucose in your bloodstream will drop significantly. This is because your diet will be low in carbohydrates. In response to this, your body will stimulate the liver to break down the carbohydrates that are stored there in the form of glycogen. This will then temporarily increase the glucose levels in the bloodstream.

However, this is not sustainable in the long run. The blood sugar levels will soon fall once again. It is at this point that the body will release a hormone known as the cortisol hormone. In other words, this hormone is referred to as the stress hormone as it is usually released at the point at which the body is in distress.

The main function of the cortisol hormone is to increase your energy levels so as to support the normal functioning of the body organs. This is usually achieved by stimulating the liver cells to break down the glycogen and protein in the body to produce glucose. While in this state, the body will reduce its energy requirements so as to conserve energy.

The release of the cortisol hormone is, therefore, one of the key factors that are responsible for the keto flu that is experienced within the first few days of the ketogenic diet. Many people will report feeling cold, especially in their extremities due to the slowdown in the body's processes. Others may report experiencing brain fog and mental fatigue due to the same reasons.

To reduce the stress levels that are caused by the cortisol hormone, you are advised to get adequate rest. This measure is very important as it reduces the cortisol levels in your system, lessening some of the keto flu symptoms. You are generally advised to aim for about 7 to 8 hours of sleep every night.

In addition, you are encouraged to keep your body hydrated all day. Water is very important in keeping some of the signs and symptoms of the keto fuel in control. You are advised to take a minimum of eight glasses of water per day. However, this could greatly vary depending on your current body weight.

Thyroid Issues

The thyroid is a small organ that is found at the base of the neck. The hormone is responsible for the production of hormones that regulate the rate of metabolism in the body. Some of the other functions of the thyroid include regulating reproductive health, immunity, mood, and maintaining the body temperature.

In order to function properly, the thyroid needs glucose so as to produce the hormones that are responsible for the above-named functions. When the levels of carbohydrates are low, as is the case in the ketogenic diet, the glucose levels in the bloodstream drop significantly. This significantly affects the thyroid gland which is heavily reliant on glucose. As a result, the production of hormones will slow down and people who have hypothyroidism are likely to experience worse symptoms.

At this point, you may wonder, aren't the ketones a sufficient form of fuel for the thyroid? Well, it is rather unfortunate that the ketogenic diet does not supply the right form of energy that is required to keep the thyroid functioning optimally.

To reduce the stress that is caused by the low glucose levels as well as the low thyroid function, you are advised to make sure that your diet contains the right kind of carbohydrates. It is true that the thyroid gland requires a given level of glucose in order to function properly. However, this does not mean that the thyroid gland requires you to eat foods that are highly processed or rich in calories. It all boils down to the quality of the carbohydrates that you are eating.

Refined and processed carbohydrates such as sugar, grains, and flour should strictly be avoided. Instead, you should opt for healthy carbohydrates found in fruits, vegetables, nuts, and seeds. The amount of carbohydrates that you will need for the proper functioning of the thyroid will generally vary from one individual to the next depending on factors such as age, gender, weight, and pre-existing thyroid problems.

You are also encouraged to supplement your diet using vitamins and minerals. Before you do this, you will need to visit a doctor to determine the vitamins and minerals that you will need to supplement. This is usually determined by carrying out different blood tests. In addition, your medical practitioner should advise you on the brands and dosages that you will need to take care of your thyroid issues. Some of the common minerals that get affected by thyroid problems include magnesium, vitamin D3, zinc, and selenium, among many others.

Adrenal Fatigue

Adrenal fatigue refers to a collection of signs and symptoms which are associated with chronic stress or some specific infections. These symptoms include fatigue, brain fog, sleep disorders, digestive problems, and skin discoloration among many other symptoms.

The adrenal glands are responsible for the production of a wide variety of hormones which are important for our biological processes. While the cause of adrenal fatigue is still a subject under research, many scientists claim that it is caused by chronic stress.

This stress could either be external or internal. While on the ketogenic diet, the body is usually subjected to some form of stress due to the low levels of glucose in the blood. This stress is sufficient to cause an overproduction of the cortisol hormone, leading to adrenal fatigue.

The main step that you can take to reduce the stress that is caused by adrenal fatigue is to adopt a diet that is friendly to the thyroid. This will keep the thyroid and adrenal glands from over-working themselves.

Chapter 8: Gut Health

Gut Complications while on the Ketogenic Diet

It has been scientifically proven that cutting out certain foods from your diet will create an imbalance in your digestive system. The transition to the new ratio of nutrients in the ketogenic diet is no exception. Many people will, therefore, experience diarrhea, constipation, painful cramping, and even increased flatulence and bloating.

The drastic reduction in the intake of carbohydrates and the increase in the intake fats is one of the factors that cause digestive problems when you first begin the ketogenic diet. This is because fats usually require a lot of energy for them to be broken down into ketone bodies. The metabolism of some people may not be adapted to this type of activity. As such, the body may not be able to utilize the fats consumed, and most of this fat will most likely be expelled in the form of stool, hence the diarrhea.

The gut cells also feed off short-chain fatty acids which are usually found in fruits, vegetables, and grains, which are all greatly restricted while on the ketogenic diet. As such, the gut cells will need to take some time to adjust to the new meal plan, during which you are likely to experience the above mentioned digestive problems.

The inadequate consumption of fiber could also responsible for the constipation that takes places when you first begin the diet. Fiber is important for the proper functioning of the gut. Hence, when the intake of fiber is restricted as is the case with the ketogenic diet, you are likely to experience some digestive problems.

Remedies to Gut Complications

As a remedy, you could increase your consumption of foods that are rich in fiber and which are still allowed on the ketogenic diet. Some of these foods include nuts, seeds, leafy greens such as spinach, and cruciferous vegetables. You are advised to avoid fiber supplements as these are usually high in carbohydrates and could bring about an imbalance in your intake of nutrients while on the ketogenic diet.

In addition, water is quite literally a solution to most if not all of the problems that you will experience while on the ketogenic diet. If your body is adequately hydrated, digested food will be to pass through the gut smoothly, reducing the occurrence of constipation. In addition, an increase in the intake of water will reduce the presence of gas in your stomach, reducing the feeling of being bloated.

You will also need to reduce your consumption of coconut products and other foods that contain medium-chain triglycerides (MCTs). These fats are highly encouraged for the ketogenic diet as they are considered to be healthy fats. These MCTs are usually digested very quickly. This is a good thing as it encourages the release of ketones and consequently leads to an increase in the amount of energy available to the body. However, because of how fast the MCT oils are digested, consuming high levels of foods that are rich in these oils could cause severe abdominal cramps and diarrhea.

To reduce the effect of the MCT oils, you are advised to ease up on the consumption of these foods and supplements. You could also give your body sufficient time to fully ease into the diet.

In some situations, some people report feeling like the food they consume is sitting in the stomach for too long. This usually has the effect of leaving you feeling constantly full and bloated. If you experience this, you are advised to increase your intake of probiotic foods and supplements. Probiotic foods usually contain a high amount of digestive enzymes which encourage the breakdown of food to release energy.

Chapter 9: Wellness and Longevity

So far, you must admit that the ketogenic diet has plenty of benefits apart from weight loss. It is exactly because of these additional benefits that this diet has grown in popularity across the globe. Can you imagine losing weight while improving your general health and well- being? I know it must sound unbelievable, but really, it is not. In this chapter, we will dive deep into some of the benefits that the ketogenic has to offer, making sure to critically explain the scientific research that has been published to support these claims.

An extended lifespan. According to new research that was published by the Harvard T.H. Chan School of Public Health, the ketogenic diet – through the process of dietary and calorie restriction is believed to alter the mitochondrial networks inside the energy-producing cells, increasing lifespan and promoting good health.

Generally, the mitochondria – the energy-producing cells exist in networks that are constantly changing their shape, depending on the energy demands of an individual. Their capacity to constantly change however generally declines with age. As such, a causal relationship has been established between the dynamic changes of the shape of the mitochondria cells and longevity. This study, therefore, proved the importance of the elasticity of the mitochondria for the benefits of the ketogenic diet, particularly longevity.

Protection from diabetes and hypertension. The ketogenic diet is a high-fat, moderate-protein, and low-carb diet. As such, when you first begin the ketogenic diet, the amount of carbohydrates that you will be consuming will definitely be less than what you were consuming before.

Because of this, the levels of glucose in your bloodstream will drop significantly.

When this happens, the body will go into a state of distress characterized by an increase in the production of the cortisol hormone. This hormone will stimulate the breakdown of the glycogen stored in the liver as well as the breakdown of protein to produce glucose. When this happens, the levels of insulin will initially rise significantly so as to facilitate the uptake of glucose by the cellular structures in the body.

However, once the body becomes keto adapted, the insulin levels in the blood will gradually drop, facilitating fat burning. The drop in insulin consequently leads to a drop in blood sugar levels. This reduces the occurrence of insulin resistance as the insulin available in the body is able to facilitate the uptake of insulin to the different cellular structures. This is important as it decreases the risk of type 2 diabetes. Type 2 diabetes is a chronic condition in which the body becomes resistant to insulin or is unable to produce insulin.

Improved heart health and protection from cardiovascular disease. A drop in insulin levels also leads to an increase in the breakdown of body fat, facilitating the use of fat as an energy source. This greatly reduces the cholesterol levels in the body, and cases of obesity and cardiovascular diseases. Insulin is a hormone that signals the liver and other cellular structures to take in glucose from the bloodstream. Insulin, therefore, facilitates the use of glucose as a source of energy. Low levels of insulin, therefore, reduce the use of glucose as a source of energy, forcing the body to turn to the breakdown of fat as an alternative source of energy.

Insulin is a major hormone that is produced by the pancreas. In addition, insulin is one of the major hormones in the human body. Elevated levels of insulin are believed to cause hormonal imbalance of some of the female sex hormones – estrogen and progesterone. However, with the ketogenic diet, the insulin levels in the body drop significantly, restoring hormonal imbalance to the female body in particular.

The hormone estrogen stimulates an increase in the production of HDL cholesterol, which is considered to be the good type of cholesterol and a decrease in the production of LDL which is the harmful type of cholesterol. This is very important as it prevents the accumulation of LDL cholesterol in the heart chambers and in the blood vessels, reducing the risk of heart failure among other heart complications.

The hormone also promotes the relaxation and dilation of blood vessels which promotes the flow of blood in the body. This ensures that all body parts receive sufficient amounts of oxygen and nutrients which are needed for survival. It also enhances the blood clot formation process. A drop in the estrogen levels in the bloodstream leads to an increase in HDL cholesterol, which leads to a buildup of fat in the blood vessels, increasing the risk of developing a heart attack or even stroke, which are common symptoms in menopausal women.

Improvement in insulin sensitivity. To understand the concept of increased insulin sensitivity, you will first need to understand the role that insulin plays in the digestive system. As we mentioned before, insulin is a hormone that is responsible for the uptake of glucose into the cellular structures. Whenever you eat, the food enters the digestive system where it is broken down into different nutrients. These nutrients are then absorbed into the bloodstream where they are transported to different organs for nourishment.

When starchy foods are broken down in the gut, glucose is released. Glucose is the primary source of energy for the body. Hence, once the glucose is absorbed into the bloodstream, it is transported to the liver, the brain, and all other body organs where it is needed for energy.

The pancreas is usually responsible for the production of the insulin hormone which is responsible for the absorption of glucose from the bloodstream and into the cellular structures. We, therefore, see that insulin plays a critical role in regulating blood sugar levels. In the absence of insulin, glucose will most likely accumulate in the bloodstream leading to the condition known as Diabetes. However, in the event that the cellular structures in the body are unable to respond to insulin to take up the glucose in the bloodstream, then we have a condition known as insulin resistance.

When the cells in the liver and other body organs are unable to absorb the glucose in the blood, the blood sugar levels continue to rise as more glucose accumulates in the blood. The pancreas then responds to this by producing even higher amounts of insulin to deal with the increasing amount of blood sugar floating in the bloodstream.

While the pancreas can keep up with the production of high amounts of insulin for a short duration of time, it most certainly cannot keep up with this production for long. As such, the pancreatic cells will get damaged, and the glucose levels in the blood will become abnormally high. At this point, an individual will find that they have both high blood sugar levels and high insulin levels.

Insulin resistance is actually considered to pre-diabetes. This is because if there are no changes to your diet and pancreas, then you may not be able to keep up with all the blood sugar that is circulating in your bloodstream and you will be diagnosed with type 2 diabetes.

Since the ketogenic diet is a very low-carb diet, the levels of glucose in your body system are expected to gradually decrease as your body becomes adapted to the ketogenic diet. While the levels of insulin are initially expected to rise within the first few days or even weeks of the ketogenic diet, the insulin levels gradually decline as the body is forced to utilize the alternative source of fuel produced from the breakdown of fat reserves.

As a result of the decreased insulin levels in the bloodstream, the cells become more sensitive to any insulin released into the bloodstream. As such, it does not accumulate within the blood. Instead, it is utilized during the uptake of ketones by the different cellular structures in the body.

Retarded growth of tumors. The ketogenic diet leads to a decrease in the growth of cancerous tumors and increased sensitivity to chemotherapy. When cancerous cells are exposed to environments that contain lower glucose levels, proliferation, and cell death quickly follow. This is a process known as cell starvation.

Since the ketogenic diet is a low-carb diet, some scientists believe that the low glucose environment can starve the cancer cells by preventing them from using glucose for cellular growth and development. There is however no concrete evidence that the ketogenic diet will indeed benefit the cancer patients. However, there are clinical trials that are currently on going.

One of the main stumbling blocks to the use of the ketogenic diet to cure cancer is that the ketogenic diet is a challenging diet that requires a lot of discipline in order to stick to the diet and a lot of patience in waiting for the results. Cancer patients may not have the ability to stick to this diet as it may lead to unintentional weight loss which may leave them further malnourished. Even though cancer patients may master the discipline that is required to stick to this diet, they may not have the strength to go through the physical and psychological discomfort that comes with the keto flu.

Reduced inflammation. Inflammation is a common symptom of all chronic diseases that we face today. It is known to occur whenever the body is trying to heal itself. However, whenever inflammation occurs for too long, it is associated with some negative effects.

A ketogenic diet involves increased consumption of foods that are rich in fats and oils. These high fats and oils decrease the production of Leukotriene B4 (LTB4) which is involved in various cellular processes that are related to inflammation. In addition, through the ketogenic diet, we have a significant decrease in inflammatory markers such as cytokines and C-reactive protein.

Improved brain functionality and cognitive functions. The ketogenic diet, just like exercising, leads to the production of a protein called brain-derived neurotrophic factor (BDNF) within the nerve cells. This protein is especially important in learning, memory, and production of new nerve cells in the hippocampus.

In addition, while on the ketogenic diet, people mainly rely on the use of ketone bodies as opposed to glucose due to the low-carb and high-fat nature of the diet. Ketone bodies are believed to be a much more powerful source of energy for the brain leading to increased brain functionality.

Ketones are also believed to be a much more efficient source of energy as compared to glucose. This is because ketones reduce the amount of destructive free radicals that are produced by the brain. This is significant as it reduces oxidative stress on the brain as well as the other body organs. This improves mental performance and keeps the brain from aging.

Ketones are responsible for increasing the production of GABA, gamma-aminobutyric acid, which is the main neurotransmitter in the body. By increasing the production of GABA, ketones can reduce the number of neurons that are actively firing in the brain, improving your ability to focus. This is also believed to reduce anxiety and stress.

Ketone bodies also reduce the number of free radicals – extra neurons that are firing in the brain. This is achieved by improving the efficiency and the energy levels of the mitochondria which are the powerhouse of the cell. In addition, ketosis can help you to manufacture new mitochondria and to increase ATP in your brain's memory cells. This is very important in improving your memory.

The ketogenic diet is also very important to people with neurodegenerative disorders such as epilepsy, Parkinson's disease, and Alzheimer's disease. These disorders are usually characterized by the brain's inability to utilize the available glucose to handle cognition and perception. The ketogenic diet, therefore, comes in to provide an alternative source of energy which is actually more potent than glucose.

In addition, most of our brain tissue is made up of fatty acids. Hence, since the ketogenic diet is high in fats and oils, it provides the brain with omega-3 and omega-6 which are very important for the proper functioning of the brain. This, in turn, has a positive impact on the proper learning and execution of an individual.

Chapter 10: Everything you need to know about Beginning the Ketogenic Diet

Now that you know all there is to know about the ketogenic diet and especially how it applies to women, I bet you are probably planning your meal plan so that you can start the diet. However, hold your horses! There's just one more thing remaining before you can go ahead to start the diet. You need to be aware of what to expect when you begin the diet. As the adage goes, knowledge is power, and it is not an exception in this context. You will need to be aware of what to expect when you begin the diet so that you are better prepared to handle any situations that may come up in the course of the diet.

Weight loss: Although the ketogenic diet has a myriad of benefits to offer to its users, the main reason why you have decided to take up this diet is probably that you have heard or read about how the ketogenic diet is efficient in weight loss. As such, once you begin the diet, one of your main expectations will be to lose weight.

As you know by now, the ketogenic diet is low in carbohydrates, moderate in protein, and high in fats. This implies that the intake of simple sugars and starch is greatly reduced forcing the body to find an alternative source of energy. The body then shifts from breaking down glucose to breaking down stored fats to generate energy for the body functions. Hence, once the body is fully in the state of ketosis, it utilizes ketones as opposed to glucose as the main source of energy, leading to weight loss.

However, you need to be aware that within the first few days and probably even the first month, the weight loss will be as a result of the loss of water content in the body. When you cut down your intake of carbohydrates, your body will begin by breaking down the carbohydrates stored in the liver. These carbohydrates usually hold on to a lot of water. Hence, when they are broken down, the water content will be released and excreted in the form of urine. This will then result in weight loss through the loss of water content. It is once you ease into the diet and begin to break down fats that you will then experience weight loss through the loss of fat content.

In some situations, you may experience weight gain as opposed to weight loss while on the ketogenic diet. There are several reasons why this could occur. However, the main reason could be that you are feeding on high calorie fats, proteins, or carbohydrates which are causing the weight gain. As you know by now, any time you eat more calories than those needed by your body, you should expect some weight gain. To prevent this from happening, you could download a calorie-tracking application to help you keep track of your caloric intake from each of the three major food groups.

In some cases, severely limiting your intake of calories could slow down your metabolic rate, reducing the rate at which you break down your food to produce energy. When this occurs, most of the food that you consume will be stored in the liver and in other body organs as fat, leading to weight gain. You are advised to always keep in mind that while the ketogenic diet is about calorie restriction, it is not starvation. As such, you must always ensure that your body receives all the macro and micronutrients that it requires for proper functioning. This can be done by downloading an application to track your intake of food to ensure you are not severely starving yourself.

In the event that you are not consuming too much of any food group or severely limiting your calorie intake, then it could be that your body is not fully in the state of ketosis. You could refer in the earlier chapters to determine the signs that inform you whether or not your body has achieved the state of ketosis. In this case, your body will still be burning the starch to produce energy and the fats you consume will simply be stored in the body, leading to weight gain. If this is the case, you should go back to the drawing board to ensure that your diet actually fits the description of the standard ketogenic diet.

The keto flu: Under normal circumstances, fat is usually reserved as a secondary source of energy with carbohydrates being the primary source of energy. During ketosis, the body usually switches from using glucose to using ketone bodies as the primary source of energy. This situation mainly occurs when the body is undergoing starvation or fasting. Hence, when you first adopt the very low-carb diet that is the ketogenic diet, you are most likely going to experience some withdrawal-like symptoms due to the reduced intake of carbohydrates.

The transition to the ketogenic diet can be especially difficult for most people. It is usually characterized by some signs and symptoms, collectively known as the keto flu. While these signs and symptoms occur in most people, some people go through the transition process without any side effects. They include nausea, vomiting, constipation, dizziness, weakness, poor concentration, irritability, muscle cramps, difficulty in sleeping, stomach pain, and cravings. The severity of these symptoms, however, varies from one person to the next.

People generally experience these side effects in the first week of the ketogenic diet. However, in some cases, these symptoms may occur for more than one week. Due to the severity of these symptoms, some people may throw in the towel at this point, vowing to themselves that the diet does not work. However, now that you know that it is just a phase, it is my hope that you will hold on just a little longer, keeping in mind that the beginning is definitely the hardest part of the entire process.

The good news is that these signs and symptoms are to a large extent actually manageable using different home remedies and lifestyle changes. Below are some of the measures that you can put in place to manage the flu-like symptoms and to make the transition easier for you. They are:

Hydration: It is difficult to fully stress the importance of water during the ketogenic diet as it has a myriad of benefits for your body. Before we state the benefits, you must remember that in the first few days of the ketogenic diet, the body will break down the carbohydrates stored in the liver to produce energy. These carbohydrates which are usually stored as glycogen usually bind themselves to water. Hence, during the break down of glycogen, water will also be broken down and excreted through different ways. It, therefore, becomes important to replenish your water supply through constant hydration. This will then reduce the symptoms of fatigue and muscle cramping that are associated with the keto flu.

Eating enough fat: People who begin the ketogenic diet usually report increased cravings for pastries such as cookies, bread and bagels, sugary foods, and other high-carb foods. To reduce the occurrence of these cravings, you should make sure that you are actually eating enough fat as per the ketogenic diet. Eating enough fat will reduce the occurrence of hunger pangs and cravings and will keep you satisfied for longer durations of time.

Get adequate sleep: Fatigue and irritability are some of the common symptoms of the keto flu. To reduce these symptoms, you should make sure that you are having adequate sleep. Some of the measures that you can put in place to make sure that you actually get adequate sleep include reducing your coffee intake, taking a bath before, and cutting out light to make sure that you have a dark environment which is conducive for sleep.

Avoid heavy exercise: In as much as physical activity is very important for your general health and well-being, you are advised to stick to light exercises or to avoid exercising all together until you are fully adapted to the ketogenic diet. Some of the exercises that you should engage in include walking, yoga, and leisurely cycling. This will go a long way in reducing the symptoms of fatigue, stomach pain, and muscle cramps that are associated with the keto flu.

Mental fogginess: Mental clarity and improved performance are believed to be the benefits of the ketogenic diet. However, this only occurs once the body is fully into the state of ketosis and adapted to the use of ketones as a source of energy. You should, therefore, expect some form of mental fogginess once you begin the ketogenic diet.

Mental fogginess, also known as brain fog, usually occurs within the first few weeks of the ketogenic diet, after which this symptom completely disappears. When you begin the ketogenic diet, the amount of carbohydrates that you will be consuming will decrease significantly. This implies that there will be a decrease in the circulation of glucose in the body. After a few days of the ketogenic diet, the body will turn on the power-saving mode due to the increased stress levels caused by the decrease in glucose. Before the body actually begins to break down the fat reserves in the body to produce ketone bodies in satisfactory amounts, most people will report experiencing brain fatigue.

However, once the body increases its production of ketones to a satisfactory amount and adapts to the use of ketones as an alternative source of energy, many people will experience increased mental clarity and performance. This is because the ketone bodies are a much more powerful source of energy as compared to glucose.

The effects of the mental fogginess should disappear within a couple of weeks or even within a month depending on an individual. However, it is generally believed that the effects of mental fogginess should disappear any time after your body enters ketosis to the time you become fully adapted to the use of ketones.

In the event that you are still experiencing mental fogginess, or the symptoms of brain fog are getting worse after a month of being on the ketogenic diet, then it is about time that you visit your medical doctor for consultation. Prolonged mental fatigue could be a result of a mineral deficiency or could be a symptom of another condition.

Digestive problems: As you know, cutting out certain foods from your diet will definitely create an imbalance in your digestive system. The transition to the new ratio of nutrients in the ketogenic diet is no exception. Many people will therefore experience diarrhea, constipation, painful cramping, and even bloating.

The drastic reduction in the intake of carbohydrates and the increase in the intake of fats cause digestive problems when you first begin the ketogenic diet. This is because fats usually require a lot of energy for them to be broken down into ketone bodies. The metabolism of some people may not be adapted to this type of activity. As such, the body may not be able to utilize the fats consumed, and most of this fat will most likely be expelled in the form of stool, hence the diarrhea.

In addition, the gut cells usually feed off short-chain fatty acids which are usually found in fruits, vegetables, and grains, which are all restricted on the ketogenic diet. As such, the gut cells will need to take some time to adjust to the new meal plan, during which you are likely to experience the above mentioned digestive problems.

The inadequate consumption of fiber could also be responsible for the constipation that occurs when you first begin the diet. Fiber is important for the proper functioning of the gut. Hence, when the intake of fiber is restricted as is the case with the ketogenic diet, you are likely to experience some digestive problems.

As a remedy, you could increase your consumption of foods that are rich in fiber and which are still allowed on the ketogenic diet. Some of these foods include nuts, seeds, leafy greens such as spinach, and cruciferous vegetables. You are advised to avoid fiber supplements as these are usually high in carbohydrates and could bring about an imbalance in your intake of nutrients while on the ketogenic diet.

You are also advised to remain hydrated to reduce some of these digestive problems and to avoid further complications. Water will keep you hydrated despite the loss of water through the process of diarrhea. In addition, water could ease the occurrence of constipation as well as the feeling of being bloated.

Lastly, you should avoid dairy products as much as possible as dairy products are believed to cause stomach upsets, bloating, as well as other digestive problems. This implies that you should cut out all cheese, milk, cream, and other dairy products.

Keto breath: While bad breath is generally believed to come from poor dental hygiene practices, bad breath from ketosis is caused by the high-protein nature of the ketogenic diet.

While on the ketogenic diet, the body will shift into a state of ketosis where it breaks down the fats stored in the body to release ketone bodies which serve as an alternative source of fuel. Ketone bodies usually have a distinct smell which makes the breath of the dieter to be sweet and fruity. Acetone, one of the three common forms of ketone bodies, has a different smell that can be likened to the smell of nail polish remover.

Alternatively, keto breath could also be caused by the changes in the diet. The ketogenic diet is typically low in carbohydrates but high in proteins and fat. The breakdown of protein in the body leads to an increase in the production of ammonia which could cause your breath and urine to have a particularly strong smell which can be likened to the smell of a cat-litter tray.

As disgusting as this may sound, it is worth noting that the breath only lasts for a couple of weeks or until the body is fully keto adapted. It is therefore reassuring to know that the keto breath will most likely disappear on its own.

To reduce the occurrence of bad breath, you could keep your body hydrated by drinking the recommended eight glasses of water per day. This is important as it will help you to flush out the excess ketone bodies in your system which could be responsible for the keto breath.

Alternatively, you could use some natural breath fresheners to keep your breath smelling fresh. This could be through the use of breath capsules made from mint, parsley, cloves, cinnamon, or fennel seeds. As you select a breath freshener, you should make sure that it is low in calories to avoid interfering with the balance of nutrients in the ketogenic diet.

You could also opt to use the tried and tested method of practicing good oral hygiene to keep your breath fresh. This implies that you should brush your teeth, floss, and rinse with an antibacterial mouth wash at least two times a day or as often as needed. Tongue scrapping could also be important in keeping your breath fresh.

Keto rash and hair loss: The keto rash is a rare inflammatory skin condition that is characterized by an itchy red rash that primarily occurs around the upper back, chest, and abdomen and a dark brown spot that is left on the skin once the rush disappears. The condition is believed to mostly occur in Asian women.

While there is limited scientific research on the condition, there is a strong correlation between the occurrence of the rash and the process of ketosis, hence the name, the keto rash.

To reduce the effects of the keto rash, you are advised to dress in cool and comfortable clothing that will reduce the amount of sweat that you are producing. In some situations, you could even carry a portable fan to keep yourself cool during the hot weather. If possible, you could install an air conditioning system in your room to reduce sweating.

If you are really affected by the itching, you may want to reduce the amount of exercise that you do or even do something brief that does not involve heavy perspiration. As such, you are advised to engage in exercises such as brief weight lifting that do not involve heavy perspiration.

After exercising, or engaging in any activity that involves heavy sweating, you are strongly advised to take a shower to clear off the sweat from your body. This is very important as it will reduce the itchiness and soreness.

If all these home remedies fail, then you are advised to visit a medical doctor who will prescribe some antibiotics, creams, and other medication that will provide you with some temporary relief from the symptoms that you will be experiencing.

Irregular periods: When you begin the ketogenic diet, the loosening of your pants and other outfits may not be the only change that you will experience. Many women who began the ketogenic diet have reported experiencing irregular periods within the first few months of beginning the ketogenic diet. Some women have reported experiencing amenorrhea, a condition that involves the absence of the menstrual cycle for a period of three months or more. Some women have reported receiving a heavier menstrual flow while others have reported experiencing a lighter menstrual flow during the first few months of the ketogenic diet. Other women have reported experiencing their periods more frequently, implying that their menstrual cycle has been shortened.

As you are aware by now, the ketogenic diet involves the state of ketosis - where the body breaks down fats to produce ketone bodies which supply the body with energy. This diet often causes rapid weight loss within a very short period of time. Scientific research has proven that quickly losing your weight can lead to sharp drops in the level of estrogen in your bloodstream. This has the potential of causing irregular periods in most women.

The decreased levels of estrogen in the body have the potential of causing other complications to the female body. Some of these complications include vaginal dryness and reduced fertility due to the missed periods. The most worrying side effect is probably the loss of bone mass which could place you at risk of developing osteoporosis.

To resume your normal menstrual cycle while still on the ketogenic diet, you are advised to increase your intake of calories or to tone down on some of the physical activities and work outs that you have been engaging in. In his article, Dr. Throppil states that most people have a "happy weight" where their bodies will resume the normal menstrual cycle. Since this weight may not be obvious at the beginning, you are advised to take on a trial and error approach where you consciously increase the amount of calories that you consume and observe the results. This could also involve removing one or several high-intensity workouts from your fitness regime. You will be surprised that for some people, putting on some extra 5 kilograms is enough to restore their regular menstrual cycle.

I bet you are now probably wondering how long it will take for you to resume your menstrual cycle. Well, the answer is not as straight forward as you may want it to be. You will resume your regular menstrual cycle as soon as you settle into your threshold weight, what we earlier referred to as your "happy weight." This will, of course, vary from one individual to the next, depending on how fast you can get your body back to its threshold weight.

Under normal circumstances, once your body becomes fully keto-adapted, your menstrual cycle will most likely return to its regular routine. In the event that this does not happen, then it is highly likely that there are other external or internal stressors in your life which are interfering with your hormonal balance. At this point, you are advised to visit your medical practitioner for consultation.

However, it is important for you to realize that just as the ketogenic diet can make your menstrual cycle to become irregular, the diet could also make your menstrual cycle to become regular, especially if you were obese or overweight before. Weight gain has often been associated with difficulties in ovulation due to the hormonal imbalance that occurs. As such, there are some women who will resume their menstrual cycle a few weeks into the ketogenic diet. For such women, this side effect is a good thing as it will restore their hormonal balance once the threshold body weight is achieved.

Severe PMS Symptoms: The female body is believed to be highly sensitive to the smallest changes in nutrient content. This means that the significant change in nutritional content that is observed while on the ketogenic diet is likely to cause hormonal fluctuations.

When you first begin the ketogenic diet, it is highly likely that you will experience severe PMS symptoms. This is because the keto diet is essentially high in fat and low in carbohydrates. The low glucose levels in the bloodstream will stimulate the release of the cortisol hormone which is a stress hormone. The cortisol hormone will then stimulate the liver to break down glycogen in the liver and proteins to release glucose. This will result in increased levels of glucose which lead to high blood sugar. This high blood sugar will stimulate the production of high levels of insulin to encourage the cells to take up the glucose in the blood. The elevated levels of insulin will result in estrogen dominance, a condition which is a key trigger for severe PMS symptoms.

However, once your body becomes fully keto adapted, the ketogenic diet can really benefit women suffering from severe PMS symptoms and the polycystic ovarian syndrome (PCOS). This is because when done the right way, the ketogenic diet is particularly important in balancing the levels of insulin in the body. Insulin is usually responsible for regulating the blood sugar levels. When the levels of insulin are too high, they affect the female sex hormones; estrogen and progesterone. Hence, when the levels of insulin are well-regulated, we have hormonal balance in the body, resulting in less severe PMS symptoms.

Feeling cold constantly: Feeling cold is a very common and natural side effect of the ketogenic diet. This is because when the body achieves the state of ketosis, it generally tries to preserve its energy reserves as much as possible. This is done by slowing down some of the processes in the body. Hence, you will feel cold in your extremities such as your hands and feet.

If you come from the hot equatorial regions, you may not notice the cold as much. In fact, you may even appreciate the cool feeling. However, if you come from the colder regions, you may need to put in place some measures to keep yourself warm. The first measure that you could put in place could be ensuring that you drink plenty of hot drinks such as tea, coffee, chocolate, or even hot water which can help you keep warm. However, you should be cautious and avoid any high-calorie beverages as well as the dairy products. You could indulge in some hot flavored teas and coffees to keep you warm as you indulge your sweet tooth.

Alternatively, you could snuggle up! This implies that you could dress in warm and fuzzy clothing or cover yourself in heavy and warm blankets to keep you warm even as you sleep. For those who love working out, they can keep themselves warm by remaining physically active. This can be achieved by either carrying out physical work outs or keeping oneself busy in the house or at the office.

Feeling cold may also be caused by certain mineral and vitamin deficiencies in the body. For example, magnesium is an important mineral that is involved in temperature regulation. As such, if the cold feeling becomes unbearable, you could supplement your diet using various mineral supplements that are easily absorbed into the body. However, before doing this, you are advised to consult your doctor or nutritionist to carry out the necessary tests to determine the mineral deficiencies that you may have.

Mistakes to Avoid While on the Ketogenic Diet

If you are passionate about the ketogenic diet as a tool to lose weight, you have carried out all the research on how to go about the diet, and you have convinced yourself to give it a try, then there are many pitfalls that you will need to avoid if you are going to be successful. After all, it is always better to learn from the mistakes of others than to learn from your own mistakes. Below are some of the most common mistakes when it comes to the ketogenic diet:

While it is unanimously agreed upon that the ketogenic diet is hard, many people, especially women come in with this preconceived notion and end up throwing in the towel as soon as they begin. The truth of the matter is that the beginning is the hardest part. After that, it actually gets better! All you will need to do is to maintain a positive mindset and surround yourself with positive people, preferably those who share the same goals as you.

On the flip side of the coin, some other people approach the diet with a can-do mentality and end up jumping in way too fast. The problem with this is that such people will set very unrealistic goals, which will end up discouraging them altogether. As such, beginners are advised to begin with small but attainable goals which will keep them motivated. This implies that you should give yourself time to slowly ease into the diet. While doing this, remember that we are all inherently different and that life is not a competition.

Beginners who are just trying out the ketogenic diet will often put their lives on hold and exclusively focus on using the diet to lose weight. This is a mistake, as you will notice the cravings that you are feeling and get tempted to grab an unhealthy meal to satisfy your craving. Essentially, you should keep yourself busy to take your mind off your stomach until it is time to eat.

While there are many ways in which you could go about the ketogenic diet, many people often lack guidance and end up choosing a wrong plan which will only serve to stress you out and make you miserable. As I have repeated several times, the ketogenic diet is supposed to fit into your lifestyle and not the other way around. This is the only way in which you will fully ease yourself into the diet.

While on the ketogenic diet, both the quantity and quality of the food that you eat will be very important in determining the success of your diet. Due to the extreme nature of the diet, people often tend to feed on the unhealthy and fatty foods which they come across without considering the nutritional content, a habit that could easily result in weight gain. As a general rule of thumb, your food should contain healthy portions of all the macronutrients. Starches and simple sugars should, however, be minimized in order to keep the body in the state of ketosis.

People often forget to remain hydrated. People forget that it is acceptable to have beverages such as mineral water, unsweetened teas, and coffees while on the ketogenic diet. As a matter of fact, these drinks are extremely important as they help to keep hunger at bay and reduce the cravings for starchy and sweet foods.

When the time to eat comes, many people may binge eat and feast to make up for cravings that they may have experienced in between the meals. This is a mistake because binge eating will cause your blood sugar levels to sharply increase. The fluctuations in the blood sugar levels will lead to moodiness, weakness, and dizziness, which will make it harder to stick to the diet.

Some people fail to eat enough fats as per the ketogenic diet. This mainly occurs due to lack of knowledge and the fear that they will gain some weight due to the fat consumed. Many people will eat less than the required amounts. As such, the body will kick into starvation mode by cannibalizing your muscle mass and slowing down your metabolism. This will make it even more difficult to lose weight.

Some people may decide to take the whole ketogenic diet too far, making it difficult to stick to it. Essentially, methods such as the Cyclical Ketogenic Diet (CKD) and the Targeted Ketogenic Diet (TKD) are meant for beginners while the Standard Ketogenic Diet (SKD) is meant for people who are able to control their cravings in a better way. While some people may begin with the standard keto, you are strongly advised to either begin with the cyclical or targeted keto.

Due to all the rage that is associated with the ketogenic diet, many people often try out the method hoping to lose weight quickly and gain the associated benefits in record time. However, some people end up forcing the process to work so much so that they forget that weight loss is a three-part process that involves a positive mindset, a diet, and physical activity. Hence, people forget that there are many other ways of losing weight that do not necessarily involve the keto diet.

The constant, and to some extent, obsessive craving of both starchy and sugary foods is considered to be normal. However, giving in to this craving is yet another mistake that people make. People often fear that the body will waste away, and they will die from reducing their intake of carbohydrates. As such, they respond to the slightest craving by satisfying it and eventually do not gain anything from the ketogenic diet. Instead, people should try as much as possible to suppress their cravings and instead trust the process and rely on the body to produce ketones as an alternative source of fuel.

Lastly, the main factor that keeps women away from achieving their weight loss goals with the ketogenic diet is the negative publicity and comments that circulate around. Many people believe that due to the complex nature of the female body, women should keep off the diet and find alternative solutions. However, while it is true that women do have complex bodies, this is no reason to give up on the diet. All you will need to do is to educate yourself on what the ketogenic diet should be for women and be prepared for some of the side effects that may come up.

Recipe 1: Grass-Fed Burgers

Ingredients:

½ teaspoon of cumin powder

½ teaspoon of garlic powder

½ pound of ground grass-fed beef

½ pound of ground grass-fed beef liver

Sea salt

Black pepper

Desired cooking oil

Method:

1. Mix all ingredients in a bowl and form patties of your desired size.

2. Heat some cooking oil in a skillet on medium heat.

3. Cook burgers in skillet until desired doneness.

4. Store in a container in the fridge and use within 4 days.

Recipe 2: Chicken Stuffed with Bell-peppers

Ingredients:

1-pound ground chicken

4 large bell peppers, halved

1 clove garlic, minced

1 small onion, diced

1 teaspoon of paprika

1 teaspoon of chili powder

1 teaspoon of salt

½ teaspoon of freshly ground black pepper

1 cup grape tomatoes, halved

3 beaten eggs

1 tablespoon of butter

Instructions:

1. Preheat the oven to 350°F, then line a baking tray with baking sheet.

2. Next, melt the butter in a skillet over medium heat. Add the garlic, onion, salt, pepper, paprika, and chili powder, then sauté for 5 to 7 minutes.

3. Add the tomatoes and sauté for another 5 to 7 minutes.

4. Add the ground chicken and cook until golden brown or for about 15 minutes, stirring occasionally.

5. Transfer the cooked meat mixture to a medium-sized bowl and slowly mix in the eggs.

6. Lay each bell pepper half cut side up on the prepared baking sheet.

7. Pour the meat and egg mixture into the bell peppers.

8. Place the stuffed peppers in the oven and bake for 60 minutes, until the peppers soften slightly.

Recipe 3: Keto egg muffins

Ingredients:

12 eggs

2 scallions, finely chopped

140g of salami

170g of shredded cheese

Salt and pepper to taste

Instructions:

1. Preheat oven to 350° Fahrenheit, then grease a muffin pan with butter.

2. Chop up the scallions and the salami and add them to the bottom of the muffin pan.

3. In a separate bowl, whisk eggs together with seasoning and pesto. Add the cheese and mix well.

4. Next, pour egg batter on top of scallions and salami.

5. Bake for 15-20 minutes depending on the size of the muffin pan.

6. These can be prepared in a big batch ahead of time. Keep them refrigerated for 3-4 days, or freeze for longer shelf life.

Recipe 4: Grain-free Pancakes

Ingredients:

¼ cup of coconut flour

½ teaspoon of baking powder

1/4 teaspoon of salt

½ cup of whipped cream

1 egg

1 teaspoon vanilla extract

½ tablespoon of organic honey

1 tablespoon butter

Ground cinnamon

Method:

1. Preheat the skillet over medium heat.

2. In a bowl, mix the eggs, vanilla, and cream.

3. In a separate bowl, mix the coconut flour, baking soda, and salt, then gently stir the wet ingredients into the dry ingredients.

4. Melt the butter in a skillet.

5. Pour about 2 to 3 tablespoons of butter into the skillet to form pancakes that are at least 10 cm in diameter.

6. Cook the pancakes for 2 -3 minutes on each side until golden brown.

7. Repeat the process until all the batter is consumed.

Recipe 5: Vegetarian Keto Casserole

Ingredients:

½ leek

⅓ cup green olives

12 eggs

1 cup heavy whipping cream

7 oz. shredded cheese

1 tsp onion powder

3 oz. cherry tomatoes

1 oz. parmesan cheese, shredded

Salt and pepper to taste.

Instructions:

1. Preheat the oven to 400° Fahrenheit.

2. Rinse and slice the leek. Next, add the leek to a greased baking dish along with the pitted olives.

3. Add the eggs, cream, the larger bit of shredded cheese, and onion powder to a separate bowl.

4. Whisk to combine the ingredients and season them with salt and pepper.

5. Pour the mixture of egg over the olives and leeks, and then add the tomatoes and parmesan cheese over the olive mixture.

6. Bake in the oven for about 30 to 40 minutes or until golden brown on the top and firm in the middle.

Recipe 6: Grain-free Cauliflower Pizza

Ingredients:

1 pound of pizza florets

2 eggs, lightly beaten

1 teaspoon salt

1 teaspoon dried oregano

1 teaspoon garlic powder

Pizza toppings of your choice

Method:

1. Pre-heat the oven to 400◦C.

2. Place the cauliflower in a food processor and pulse it until it is finely chopped, then transfer it to a large bowl.

3. In the bowl, add the eggs, salt, oregano, and garlic powder and mix well.

4. Transfer the cauliflower mixture onto the baking sheet and spread it to form the pizza crust.

5. Bake the crust for about 20 minutes, or until the crust is slightly golden.

6. Add your desired toppings, and then bake for about 10 – 15 minutes.

Recipe 7: Low Carb Oatmeal

Ingredients:

1 cup of coconut milk or unsweetened almond milk

1 tablespoon flaxseed, whole

1 tablespoon chia seeds

1 tablespoon sunflower seeds

1 pinch salt

Instructions:

1. Mix all ingredients in a small saucepan and bring to a boil.

2. Lower the heat and let simmer until oatmeal is at desired thickness. This should only take a couple of minutes.

3. Top the mixture with butter and coconut milk – or even with almond milk and cinnamon – or fresh, unsweetened berries. The possibilities are endless.

4. You can make a bigger batch of this ahead of time and reheat it for your week ahead.

Recipe 8: Chicken Wings

Ingredients:

2 pounds chicken wings

1 tablespoon of salt

1 teaspoon of paprika

1 teaspoon of freshly ground black pepper

1 tablespoon of baking powder

1 teaspoon of garlic

2 tablespoons of coconut oil

2 tablespoons of hot sauce

Instructions:

1. Wash the chicken wings and pat dry.

2. In a small bowl, combine the salt, pepper, baking powder, paprika, and garlic.

3. Place the wings in a sealable plastic bag and add the spice mixture.

4. Seal and shake the bag to coat the wings.

5. Preheat a skillet over medium heat and melt the coconut oil in the warm pan.

6. Place the wings in the skillet and cover.

7. Cook for 10 to 12 minutes.

8. Flip the wings and cook for another 10 to 12 minutes, until golden brown.

9. Remove the wings from the heat and let cool for 5 minutes.

10. Coat the wings with hot sauce, if desired.

Recipe 9: Scrambled Eggs and Halloumi Cheese

Ingredients:

85g halloumi cheese, diced

100g bacon, diced

2 tablespoons olive oil

2 scallions

4 eggs

½ cup fresh parsley, chopped

½ cup pitted olives

Salt and pepper to taste

Instructions:

1. Slice up some halloumi cheese and bacon bits.

2. Heat the olive oil on medium-high in a frying pan and fry the halloumi, scallions, and bacon together until they are nicely browned.

3. In a bowl, mix together the parsley, eggs, salt, and pepper.

4. Place the egg mixture into the frying pan on top of the bacon and cheese bits. Turn the heat to low, add the olives and mix for a couple of minutes.

5. Serve with or without a salad.

Recipe 10: Simple Homemade bacon

Ingredients:

2 pounds pork belly

⅔ cup salt

2 tablespoons of freshly ground black pepper

Any dried herbs and spices

Instructions:

1. Remove the skin from the pork belly with a very sharp knife. As you remove it, try to keep the skin intact, in one piece.

2. Rinse the pork belly and pat dry with a kitchen towel.

3. In a small bowl, mix together the salt, pepper, and any dried herbs and spices.

4. Rub the mixture on both sides of the pork belly.

5. Place the pork belly inside a sealed airtight container and store in the refrigerator for 5 to 7 days. The flavor becomes stronger the longer you cure it.

6. Flip the pork belly over every day. (Make sure you wash your hands thoroughly before touching the pork belly.)

7. After 5 to 7 days, remove the pork belly from the refrigerator, and rinse off the salt, pepper, and any other herbs and spices. Pat dry.

8. Preheat the oven to 200°F (90°C).

9. Place a roasting rack in a roasting pan. Place the pork belly fat side up on the rack.

10. Bake until the meat reaches an internal temperature of 150°F. This usually takes about an hour and a half to two hours.

11. Remove the pork belly from the oven and let it cool for 30 minutes.

12. Wrap the meat in parchment paper, and store in the refrigerator overnight or for 12 hours.

Recipe 11: Classic Bacon and Eggs

Ingredients:

4 eggs

140g bacon, in slices

Cherry tomatoes

Fresh parsley

Instructions:

1. Fry the bacon in a pan on medium-high heat until crispy.

2. Put aside cooked bacon on a plate. Leave the bacon grease inside the pan.

3. Use this same bacon grease pan to fry the eggs.

4. Place the pan over medium heat, and crack your eggs into the bacon grease.

5. You can cook the eggs any way you like to eat them. Sunnyside up eggs require that you leave the eggs to fry on one side and you cover the pan to make sure they get cooked on top. Eggs that are over easy are flipped over after a few minutes and cooked for another minute.

6. Cut the tomatoes in half and fry them at the same time as the eggs.

7. Add salt and pepper to taste.

Recipe 12: Homemade Chicken Strips

Ingredients:

1 pound of boneless chicken breasts cut into finger-like pieces

2 eggs

1 tablespoon of salt

1 teaspoon of freshly ground pepper

1 teaspoon of paprika

1 teaspoon of garlic

2 tablespoons of coconut oil

Hot sauce

Instructions:

1. Preheat the oven to 300°C, and line the baking sheet with aluminum foil.

2. Wash the chicken fingers thoroughly and pat dry using some kitchen towels.

3. In a small bowl, combine the pork rinds, salt, pepper, paprika, and garlic. Pour the mixture into a sealable bag.

4. In a larger bowl, beat the eggs and dip each fish finger into the egg wash to coat it.

5. Add the chicken breasts that are coated with the egg into the sealable bag with the spice mixture.

6. Seal the bag to allow the mixture to coat the chicken.

7. Place the chicken strips on the baking sheet and place them in the oven. Allow to bake for about 10 − 15 minutes.

Recipe 13: Tuna Cheese Melt

Ingredients:

Tuna Fish Salad

1 cup mayonnaise or sour cream

4 celery stalks

½ cup dill pickles, chopped

8 oz. tuna in olive oil

1 tsp lemon juice

1 garlic clove, minced

Salt and pepper, to taste

Toppings:

250g shredded cheese

¼ tsp cayenne pepper or paprika powder

For serving:

150g leafy greens

Olive oil

Oopsie bread (makes 6-8):

3 eggs

400g cream cheese

1 pinch salt

½ tablespoon ground psyllium husk powder

½ tsp baking powder

Instructions:

1. Preheat the oven to 350° F.

2. Mix together the salad ingredients.

3. Lay the bread slices down on a baking sheet that is lined with parchment paper. Spread the tuna mix over the bread and sprinkle some more cheese on top.

4. Add some paprika powder or cayenne pepper.

5. Bake in an oven until the cheese has turned a beautiful color, which takes around 15 minutes. Serve the sandwich with some greens that are tossed with olive oil.

For the oopsie bread:

1. Preheat the oven to 300°F.

2. Separate egg yolks into one bowl and the egg whites into another bowl.

3. Add salt to the egg whites and whip them until they are stiff. The bowl should be able to be turned upside down, and the egg white will remain in place.

4. Mix together the egg yolks and the cream cheese. If you want to add the phylum seed husk and baking powder do this now. (They serve to make the Topside have a more bread-like consistency).

5. Fold the stiff egg whites into the egg yolk mixture and try to keep the air in the egg whites.

6. Place 8 oopsie pieces on a baking tray lined with parchment.

7. Bake them in the middle of the oven for about 25 minutes or until they turn golden.

Recipe 14: Chicken Curry Pie

Ingredients:

Pie crust

¾ cup almond flour

4 tablespoons sesame seeds

4 tablespoons coconut flour

1 tablespoon ground psyllium husk powder

1 teaspoon baking powder

1 pinch salt

3 tablespoons olive oil or coconut oil

1 egg

4 tablespoons water

Filling

10 oz. cooked chickens

1 cup mayonnaise

3 eggs

½ green bell pepper, finely chopped

1 tsp curry powder

½ tsp paprika powder

½ tsp onion powder

¼ tsp ground black pepper

½ cup cream cheese

1¼ cups shredded cheese

Instructions:

1. Preheat the oven to 350°F.

2. Place all the ingredients for the pie crust into a food processor for a couple of minutes, just until the dough firms up into a ball. You can also mix the dough using a fork if you prefer to do it that way.

3. Place a piece of parchment paper onto a springform pan that is no larger than 10 inches around. Grease the bottom and sides of the dish.

4. The dough must be spread into the pan. Use an oiled spatula or your fingers that are coated in oil to do this. The crust must bake for 12 to 15 minutes.

5. Combine together all the other filling ingredients, and fill the pie crust. Bake this for 35 to 40 minutes. Or until the pie color has turned a nice golden-brown.

6. Let the pie cool. Serve with a salad and light dressing.

Recipe 15: Keto Pesto Chicken Casserole

Ingredients:

25 oz. boneless chicken thighs or chicken breasts

1 oz. butter, for frying

3 oz. red pesto or green pesto

1¼ cups heavy whipping cream

3 oz. pitted olives

5 oz. feta cheese, diced

1 garlic clove, finely chopped

Salt, and pepper

Ingredients:

1. Preheat the oven to 400°F.

2. Cut the chicken thighs/chicken breasts into bite-sized pieces. Season them with salt and pepper to taste.

3. Add the butter to a large skillet and fry the chicken bits in batches on medium-high heat until they are golden-brown.

4. Mix the pesto and heavy cream together in a small bowl.

5. Mix the fried chicken pieces in a baking dish together with the olives, feta cheese, and garlic. Add the pesto to this chicken mixture.

6. Bake in the oven for 20 to 30 minutes, until the dish gets bubbly and light brown around the edges.

Recipe 16: Keto Chicken Garam Masala

Ingredients:

25 oz. chicken breasts

3 tablespoons butter or ghee

Salt

1 red bell pepper, finely diced

1¼ cups coconut cream or heavy whipping cream

1 tablespoon fresh parsley, finely chopped

For the garam masala:

1 tsp ground cumin

1 - 2 tsp coriander seed, ground

1 tsp ground cardamom (green)

1 tsp turmeric, ground

1 tsp ground ginger

1 tsp paprika powder

1 tsp chili powder

1 pinch ground nutmeg

Directions:

1. Preheat the oven to 400°F.
2. Mix the spices together for the garam masala.

3. Cut the chicken breasts lengthwise. Place a large skillet over medium-high heat and fry the chicken in the butter until it is golden-brown.

4. Add half of the garam masala spice mix to the pan and stir it thoroughly.

5. Season with some salt, and place the chicken and all of the juices into a baking dish.

6. Finely chop the bell pepper and add it to a bowl along with the coconut cream and the remaining half of the garam masala spice mix.

7. Pour over the chicken. Bake in the oven for about 20 minutes.

8. Garnish with parsley and serve.

Recipe 17: Keto Fish Casserole

Ingredients:

2 tablespoons olive oil

15 oz. broccoli

6 scallions

2 tablespoons small capers

1⁄6 oz. butter, for greasing the casserole dish

25 oz. white fish, in serving-sized pieces

1¼ cups heavy whipping cream

1 tablespoon Dijon mustard

1 teaspoon salt

¼ teaspoon ground black pepper

1 tablespoon dried parsley

3 oz. butter

Instructions:

1. Preheat the oven to 400°F.

2. Divide the broccoli into smaller floret heads and include the stems. Peel it with a sharp knife or a potato peeler if the stem is rough or leafy.

3. Fry the broccoli florets in oil on medium-high heat for about 5 minutes, until they are golden and soft. Season with salt and pepper to taste.

4. Add finely chopped scallions and the capers. Fry these for another 1 to 2 minutes and place the vegetables in a baking dish that has been greased.

5. Place the fish tightly in amongst the vegetables.

6. Mix the parsley, whipping cream, and mustard together. Pour this over the fish and vegetables. Top it with slices of butter.

7. Bake the fish for 20 minutes or until the fish is cooked through, and it flakes easily with a fork. Serve as is or with a tasty green salad.

Recipe 18: Oven Baked Chicken in Garlic Butter

Ingredients:

3 lbs. chickens, a whole bird

2 teaspoon sea salt

½ teaspoon ground black pepper

5⅓ oz. butter

2 garlic cloves, minced

Instructions:

1. Preheat the oven to 400°F.

2. Season the chicken with salt and pepper to taste, both inside and out.

3. The chicken must go breast side up in the baking dish.

4. Combine the garlic and butter in a saucepan over medium heat. The butter should not turn brown or burn; just melt it gently.

5. Let the butter cool down for a few minutes once it is melted.

6. Pour the garlic butter mixture all over and inside the chicken. Bake the chicken on the lower oven rack for 1 to1 ½ hours, or until internal temperature reaches 180°F. Baste it with the juices from the bottom of the pan every 20 minutes.

7. Serve with the juices and a side dish of your choice.

Recipe 19: Keto Buffalo Drumsticks and Chili Aioli

Ingredients:

2 lbs. chicken drumsticks or chicken wings

2 tablespoons olive oil or coconut oil

2 tablespoons white wine vinegar

1 tablespoon tomato paste

1 tsp salt

1 tsp paprika powder

1 tablespoon Tabasco

Butter or olive oil, for greasing the baking dish

For the chili aioli:

2/3 cup mayonnaise

1 tablespoon smoked paprika powder or smoked chili powder

1 garlic clove, minced

Instructions:

1. Preheat the oven to 450° (220°C).

2. Put the drumsticks in a plastic bag.

3. Mix the ingredients for the marinade in a small bowl and pour into the plastic bag. Shake the bag thoroughly and let it marinate for 10 minutes in room temperature.

4. Coat a baking dish with oil. Place the drumsticks in the

baking bowl and let bake for 30–40 minutes or until they are done and have turned a beautiful color.

5. Mix together mayonnaise, garlic, and chili, and serve it with the drumsticks

Recipe 20: Meatloaf Wrapped in Bacon

Ingredients:

2 tablespoons butter

1 yellow onion, finely chopped

25 oz. ground beef or ground lamb/pork

½ cup heavy whipping cream

½ cup shredded cheese

1 egg

1 tablespoon dried oregano or dried basil

1 teaspoon salt

½ teaspoon ground black pepper

7 oz. sliced bacon

1¼ cups heavy whipping cream, for the gravy

Instructions:

1. Preheat the oven to 400°F.

2. Fry the onion until it is soft but not overly browned.

3. Mix the ground meat in a bowl with all the other ingredients, minus the bacon. Mix it well, but avoid overworking it as you do not want the mixture to become dense.

4. Form the meat into a loaf shape and place it in a baking dish. Wrap the loaf completely in the bacon.

5. Bake the loaf in the middle rack of the oven for about 45 minutes. If you notice that the bacon begins to overcook before the meat is done, cover it with some aluminum foil and lower the heat a bit since you do not want burnt bacon.

6. Save all the juices that have accumulated in the baking dish from the meat and bacon. They will be used to make the gravy. Mix these juices and the cream in a smaller saucepan for the gravy.

7. Bring it to a boil and lower the heat and let it simmer for 10 to 15 minutes until it has the right consistency and is not lumpy.

8. Serve the meatloaf with freshly-boiled broccoli or some cauliflower with butter, salt, and pepper.

Recipe 21: Keto Lasagna

Ingredients:

2 tablespoons olive oil

1 yellow onion

1 garlic clove

20 oz. ground beef

3 tablespoons tomato paste

½ tablespoon dried basil

1 teaspoon salt

¼ teaspoon ground black pepper

½ cup water

Keto pasta

8 eggs

10 oz. cream cheese

1 tsp salt

5 tablespoons ground psyllium husk powder

Cheese topping

2 cups crème fraiche or sour cream

5 oz. shredded cheese

2 oz. grated parmesan cheese

½ teaspoon salt

¼ teaspoon ground black pepper

½ cup fresh parsley, finely chopped

Instructions:

1. Start with the ground beef mixture. You can prepare this a day or two before you want to use it for added flavor.

2. Peel and finely chop the onion and the garlic. Fry them in olive oil until they are soft. Add the ground beef to the onion and garlic and cook until it is golden. Add the tomato paste and remaining spices.

3. Stir the mixture thoroughly and add some water. Bring it to a boil, turn the heat down, and let it simmer for at least 15 minutes, or until most of the water has evaporated. The lasagna sheets used don't soak up as much liquid as regular ones, so the mixture should be quite dry.

4. Meanwhile, make the lasagna sheets according to the instructions below.

5. Preheat the oven to 300°F.

6. Add the eggs, cream cheese, and the salt to a mixing bowl and blend into a smooth batter. Continue to whisk this while adding in the ground psyllium husk powder, just a little bit at a time. Let it sit for a few minutes to rest.

7. Using a spatula, spread the batter onto a baking sheet that is lined with parchment paper. Place more parchment paper on top and flatten it with a rolling pin until the mixture is at least 13" x 18". You can also divide it into two separate batches and use a different baking sheet for even thinner lasagna.

8. Let the pieces of parchment paper stay in place. Bake the pasta for about 10 to12 minutes. Let it cool and remove the paper. Slice into sheets that fit your baking dish.

9. Preheat the oven to 400°F. Mix the shredded cheese with sour cream and the Parmesan cheese. Reserve one or two tablespoons of the cheese aside for the topping. Add salt and pepper for taste, and stir in the parsley.

10. Place the lasagna sheets and pasta sauce in layers in a greased baking dish.

11. Spread the crème fraiche mixture and the reserved Parmesan cheese on top.

12. Bake the lasagna in the oven for around 30 minutes or until the lasagna has a nicely browned surface. Serve with a green salad and a light dressing.

Recipe 22: Green Smoothie

Ingredients:

1 avocado

1 cup of coconut milk

1 handful of berries

1 cup of spinach or kale

1 cup of chia seeds

Method:

Place all the ingredients in a blender and blend till you achieve the desired consistency.

Recipe 23: Nut and Berry Parfait

Ingredients

6 crushed almonds

6 crushed walnuts

10 diced strawberries

1/3 cup blackberries

1/3 cup raspberries

½ tablespoon chia seeds

1 teaspoon cinnamon

1 teaspoon pure vanilla extract

½ cup heavy whipping cream

Method:

1. Place the whipping cream in a bowl and add the vanilla extract.

2. Use a hand mixer on medium and whip the whipped cream for about 2 to 3 minutes, or until stiff peaks form.

3. Stir the nuts and berries into the whipped cream.

4. Add in the chia seeds and sprinkle some cinnamon on the top.

Recipe 24: Salmon and vegetables

Salmon is a type of fish that is rich in omega 3 oils, which are healthy fats that are nutritious.

Ingredients:

1 pound of salmon

2 tablespoons of lemon juice

2 tablespoons of ghee4 cloves of garlic

Method:

1. Preheat the oven to 400∘C.

2. In a bowl, mix the lemon juice, ghee, and finely diced garlic.

3. Place the salmon in a foil and pour the above mixture over it.

4. Wrap the salmon in the foil and place it in a baking sheet.

5. Bake in the oven for 15 minutes or until the salmon is cooked. You could also roast your vegetables in a separate baking sheet or alongside the salmon.

Recipe 25: Cinnamon Roll Fat Bombs

Ingredients:

1 teaspoon cinnamon

1 tablespoon coconut oil

2 tablespoons almond butter

½ cup coconut cream

Method:

1. Mix the cinnamon and the coconut cream.

2. Line a suitable baking pan with parchment paper, and spread the cinnamon and coconut cream mixture.

3. Mix ½ a teaspoon of cinnamon with coconut oil and almond butter and spread over the first layer in the baking pan.

4. Freeze for about 10 minutes, then cut into the desired squares or circular pieces.

Recipe 26: Keto Avocado Quiche

Ingredients:

Pie crust

¾ cup almond flour

4 tablespoons sesame seeds

4 tablespoons coconut flour

1 tablespoon ground psyllium husk powder

1 teaspoon baking powder

1 pinch salt

3 tablespoons olive oil or coconut oil

1 egg

4 tablespoons water

Filling

2 ripe avocados

1 cup mayonnaise

3 eggs

2 tablespoons fresh cilantro, finely chopped

1 red chili pepper, finely chopped

½ teaspoon onion powder

¼ teaspoon salt

½ cup cream cheese

1¼ cups shredded cheese

Instructions:

1. Preheat the oven to 350° F. Mix all the ingredients together for the pie dough in a food processor until the dough forms into a ball. This takes a few minutes usually. Use your hands or a fork in the absence of a food processor to knead the dough together.

2. Place a piece of parchment paper to a springform pan, no larger than 12 inches around. The springform pan makes it easier to take the pie out when it is done. Grease the pan and the parchment paper.

3. Using an oiled spatula or oil coated fingers, spread the dough into the pan. Bake the crust for 10 to 15 minutes.

4. Split the avocado in half. Remove the peel and pit it, and dice the avocado.

5. Take the seeds out from the chili and chop the chili very finely. Combine the avocado and the chili in a bowl and mix them together with the other ingredients.

6. Pour the mixture into the pie crust and bake it for 35 minutes or until it is light golden brown. Let it cool for a few minutes, and serve it with a green salad.

Conclusion

Thank you again for buying this book and sticking with it to the end!

I hope this book was able to help you to understand how the ketogenic diet can be used to lose weight and live a healthier lifestyle. In addition, I hope that the book has shed sufficient light on the ketogenic diet, specifically for women. In the process, I hope you have come to better understand yourself as a woman.

So far, I hope you have come to understand that the ketogenic diet is not merely a diet, but a way of life that comes with numerous health benefits for you. It is also my hope that you have come to appreciate the benefits that come with the ketogenic diet and have come to terms with the fact that it is not as extreme as people make it sound. In addition to the known benefits, you must be aware that the ketogenic diet is still a new concept and that there are many more benefits that are still being explored and studied by nutritionists and medical practitioners.

In as much as intermittent fasting and the ketogenic diet are perfect compliments in the weight loss journey, do not feel pressured to adopt both the methods since they still work perfectly when used independently. It is advisable that you begin with the ketogenic diet, then gradually incorporate the intermittent fasting method once you believe in yourself.

If you have started the ketogenic diet and it feels uncomfortable at first, I would advise you to give yourself time to adjust. There is no standard duration of time that it will take you to adjust to the diet, as we are all inherently different and unique. Hence, simply monitor your body and understand some of the signals that it will be communicating to you.

Throughout the whole process, you must bear in mind that the ketogenic diet will indeed test your discipline and willpower in ways that you cannot imagine or believe to be possible. However, here's a piece of encouragement; the beginning is the hardest part, and then it gets better! All you will need to do is to maintain a positive mindset and surround yourself with positive people, preferably those who share the same goals as you. In no time at all, you will find yourself able to go for longer hours of time without experiencing any cravings.

To keep yourself motivated, you could maintain a record of your feeding habits and physical activities in a spreadsheet to help you to monitor your progress and to establish any trends that could provide opportunities for growth.

It cannot be stressed enough that the ketogenic diet is not for everyone! As such, as soon as you begin the dieting process, you will need to carefully monitor your body for any signs of weakness, dizziness, light-headedness, moodiness, or even constipation. If you observe these symptoms, you are advised to stop the diet and consult the experts on the way forward.

Anyone suffering from a health condition should be careful and consult the advice of a medical practitioner before starting the ketogenic diet. This is especially the case for people suffering from diabetes or high blood pressure. Such people should persistently monitor their blood sugar levels and blood pressure at least four times daily.

The next step is to implement everything that you have learned from this book. Feel free to make any amendments and modifications to suit you and your lifestyle. After all, you must always remember that the ketogenic diet is meant to fit into your life and not the other way around.

Bearing in mind that knowledge is power, you should never stop reading, researching, or consulting experts regarding the ketogenic diet. Feel free to get the opinions of other people and frequently compare notes with them to stay motivated and optimistic. As such, now that you have successfully completed this book, start researching on the next book that you will be picking up.

Once you have gotten comfortable with the ketogenic diet, you could slowly begin to incorporate a workout or fitness program to keep yourself physically fit. Due to the intensity of the program, you will need to only consider activities that are either light or moderate. To get the most out of your fitness program, you could consult a fitness expert who will create a workout plan for you.

In conclusion, you should always bear in mind that you are a social creature, and like all social creatures, you have social needs and demands. Hence, do not avoid going to celebrations or feasts because you are on a diet. Occasionally, give yourself a break and join other people to make merry. Later, you could compensate for this by fasting for given durations of time or reducing your overall intake until you have sufficiently compensated.

Before you go

Once again I would like to remind you to join get your free report by clicking the link below

The 7 Foods you need to avoid for a successful keto journey

If you feel like you need a little extra support I would like to invite you to join my free facebook accountability group to have full access to myself so I can help you along the journey. Just type in **Keto conquer 101; learn to win the weight loss game** into the facebook search engine

Instagram- Effortless_Weightloss

Go to www.vipketoreport.com to get your Free Report, The 7 keto foods you need to avoid

References

(n.d.). Retrieved from https://helloclue.com/articles/cycle-a-z/the-immune-system-and-the-menstrual-cycle

047: David Goggins - Overcoming Obstacles, Changing Your Mindset, and How to Break Free From Your Comfort Zone. (2019, January 04). Retrieved from https://perfectketo.com/047-change-mindset/

10 Signs and Symptoms That You're in Ketosis. (n.d.). Retrieved from https://www.healthline.com/nutrition/10-signs-and-symptoms-of-ketosis#section6

16 Foods to Eat on a Ketogenic Diet. (n.d.). Retrieved from https://www.healthline.com/nutrition/ketogenic-diet-foods

16 Ways Keto for Women is Different Doesn't Need to Suck. (2018, September 26). Retrieved from http://www.wickedstuffed.com/keto-tips/keto-for-women-is-different-doesnt-need-to-suck/

5 Signs of Hormonal Imbalance. (2018, January 25). Retrieved from https://thepelvicexpert.com/blog/5-signs-hormonal-imbalance/

7-Day Ketogenic Diet Menu and Comprehensive Food List | Everyday Health. (2018, October 23). Retrieved from https://www.everydayhealth.com/diet-nutrition/ketogenic-diet/comprehensive-ketogenic-diet-food-list-follow/

A Ketogenic Diet for Beginners - The Ultimate Keto Guide. (2019, January 04). Retrieved from https://www.dietdoctor.com/low-carb/keto

Atkins, R. (1972). Dr. Atkins Diet Revolution. *Bantam edition*, 13-50.

Balanced Hormones: Why They're Important for Overall Health. (2018, June 13). Retrieved from https://nutritiouslife.com/live-consciously/balanced-hormones-health-benefits/

Biswas, C. (2018, May 25). *Diet Tips: Stylecraze*. Retrieved from Stylecraze: https://www.stylecraze.com/articles/one-meal-a-day-diet-the-ultimate-guide/#gref

Blog. (2017, August 24). Retrieved from https://koiwellbeing.com/2017/08/3-benefits-hormone-balancing-men-women/

Brooks, S. (2018, January 1). *Articles: Bulletproof*. Retrieved from Bulletproof: https://blog.bulletproof.com/keto-intermittent-fasting-weight-loss-diet/

Delauer, T. (2018, January 25). *How to Use Fasting for Inflammation and Longevity: Thomas Delauer*. Retrieved from Thomas Delauer: https://www.thomasdelauer.com/how-to-use-fasting-for-inflammation-and-longevity-benefits-of-intermittent-fasting/

Does a Ketogenic Diet Affect Women's Hormones? (2019, January 09). Retrieved from https://perfectketo.com/does-a-ketogenic-diet-affect-womens-hormones/

Does a Ketogenic Diet Affect Women's Hormones? (2019, January 09). Retrieved from https://perfectketo.com/does-a-ketogenic-diet-affect-womens-hormones/

Does keto affect cortisol levels? (n.d.). Retrieved from https://www.ruled.me/faq/does-keto-affect-cortisol-levels/

Estrogen & The Heart. (n.d.). Retrieved from https://my.clevelandclinic.org/health/articles/16979-estrogen--hormones

Female Sex Hormones: Types, Effect on Arousal, and 8 Other Functions. (n.d.). Retrieved from https://www.healthline.com/health/female-sex-hormones

Girl Talk: The Keto Diet While on Your Period. (2018, May 28). Retrieved from https://www.tasteaholics.com/news/girl-talk-the-keto-diet-while-on-your-period-16668/

Greger, M. (2004). Atkins Facts. *Latest in Human Nutrition, 2*(6), 15-23.

Gotter, A. (n.d.). Keto diet: Benefits and nutrients. Retrieved from https://www.medicalnewstoday.com/articles/319196.php

Guelpa, G., & Marie, A. (1911). La lutte contre l'épilepsie par la désintoxication et par la rééducation alimentaire. *Rev Ther Medico–Chirurgicale, 78*, 8-13.

Gunnars, K. (2016, August 16). *Nutrition: Healthline.* Retrieved from Healthline: https://www.healthline.com/nutrition/10-health-benefits-of-intermittent-fasting

Gunnars, K. (2017, June 4). *Nutrition: Healthline.* Retrieved from Healthline: https://www.healthline.com/nutrition/6-ways-to-do-intermittent-fasting

Healing Hormonal Imbalances with the Ketogenic Diet - Leanne Vogel. (2018, November 06). Retrieved from https://perfectketo.com/episode-001-leanne-vogel/

Heavy Periods: Causes & Solutions. (n.d.). Retrieved from https://flexfits.com/blogs/thefixx/heavy-periods

Hormones Do Effect the Immune System. (2016, August 04). Retrieved from https://appliedhealth.com/hormones-do-effect-the-immune-system/

Keto. (n.d.). Ketosis for Women: Does Keto Affect Female Hormones? Retrieved from https://www.kissmyketo.com/blogs/science-ketosis/ketosis-for-women-does-keto-affect-female-hormones

Keto. (n.d.). Ketosis for Women: Does Keto Affect Female Hormones? Retrieved from https://www.kissmyketo.com/blogs/science-ketosis/ketosis-for-women-does-keto-affect-female-hormones

Keto. (n.d.). Ketosis for Women: Does Keto Affect Female Hormones? Retrieved from https://www.kissmyketo.com/blogs/science-ketosis/ketosis-for-women-does-keto-affect-female-hormones

Ketogenic Diet Foods – What to Eat and to Avoid – Diet Doctor. (2019, January 04). Retrieved from https://www.dietdoctor.com/low-carb/keto/foods

Ketosis Explained: What It Is, How to Achieve It (And Why You Want To). (n.d.). Retrieved from https://perfectketo.com/guide/ultimate-guide-to-ketosis/

Ketosis: What It Is, if It's Safe, How to Achieve It, Symptoms, and More | Everyday Health. (2018, January 19). Retrieved from https://www.everydayhealth.com/diet-nutrition/ketogenic-diet/ketosis-what-it-its-safe-how-achieve-it-symptoms-more/

Ketosis: What It Is, if It's Safe, How to Achieve It, Symptoms, and More | Everyday Health. (2018, January 19). Retrieved from https://www.everydayhealth.com/diet-nutrition/ketogenic-diet/ketosis-what-it-its-safe-how-achieve-it-symptoms-more/

Lax, L. (2018, July 12). Does the Ketogenic Diet Work for Women? Retrieved from https://breakingmuscle.com/healthy-eating/does-the-ketogenic-diet-work-for-women

McIntosh, J. (2017, March 21). Ketosis: What is ketosis? Retrieved from https://www.medicalnewstoday.com/articles/180858.php

Menopause Diet: How Keto Can Help Manage Menopause Symptoms (The Best Foods To Eat). (2019, January 10). Retrieved from https://perfectketo.com/menopause-diet/

O'Hearn, L. A. (1970, January 01). The Ketogenic Diet for Health. Retrieved from http://www.ketotic.org/2014/02/the-ketogenic-diets-effect-on-cortisol.html

Okman-Kilic, T. (2015, March 04). Estrogen Deficiency and Osteoporosis. Retrieved from https://www.intechopen.com/books/advances-in-osteoporosis/estrogen-deficiency-and-osteoporosis

Person. (2018, September 14). Review on Role of Ketogenic Diet and Excessive Workout on Hormonal Imbalances in Women. Retrieved from https://www.omicsonline.org/open-access/review-on-role-of-ketogenic-diet-and-excessive-workout-on-hormonal-imbalances-in-women-2165-7904-1000373-104683.html

Polycystic Ovary Syndrome (PCOS): Symptoms, Causes, and Treatment. (n.d.). Retrieved from https://www.healthline.com/health/polycystic-ovary-disease

Rice, G. (2018, May 15). Female hormones. Retrieved from https://www.netdoctor.co.uk/healthy-living/a11666/female-hormones/

Rose, E. (2018, December 17). What to Eat on Keto: Your Complete Keto Food List. Retrieved from https://blog.bulletproof.com/keto-food-list/

Tag Archives: Insulin Resistance. (n.d.). Retrieved from http://thehormonediva.com/tag/insulin-resistance/

The Ketogenic Diet in Women. (2018, July 11). Retrieved from https://www.saragottfriedmd.com/the-ketogenic-diet-for-women/

The Ketogenic Diet in Women. (2018, July 11). Retrieved from https://www.saragottfriedmd.com/the-ketogenic-diet-for-women/

The Ketogenic Diet: A Detailed Beginner's Guide to Keto. (n.d.). Retrieved from https://www.healthline.com/nutrition/ketogenic-diet-101#other-benefits

VanHook, A. (2018, August 7). Starving Cancer Cells to Death. *Science Signaling, 11*(542).

Vogel, L. (2018, July 18). How The Keto Diet Is Different For Women. Retrieved from https://www.healthfulpursuit.com/2018/04/how-the-keto-diet-is-different-for-women/

Vogel, L. (2018, December 07). 5 Keto Diet Benefits for Women. Retrieved from https://www.healthfulpursuit.com/2018/12/res-keto-benefits-women/

Vogel, L. (2018, October 12). The Ketogenic Diet And Women's Hormones. Retrieved from https://www.healthfulpursuit.com/2018/08/ketogenic-diet-women-hormones/

Vogel, L. (2018, July 18). How The Keto Diet Is Different For Women. Retrieved from https://www.healthfulpursuit.com/2018/04/how-the-keto-diet-is-different-for-women/

What Are Hormones and What Do They Do? | Hormone Health. (n.d.). Retrieved from https://www.hormone.org/hormones-and-health/hormones/hormones-and-what-do-they-do

What Are Hormones and What Do They Do? | Hormone Health. (n.d.). Retrieved from https://www.hormone.org/hormones-and-health/hormones/hormones-and-what-do-they-do

What Is Ketosis? Why Would You Want It? And Is It Safe? – Diet Doctor. (2018, December 30). Retrieved from https://www.dietdoctor.com/low-carb/ketosis

www.ingramcontent.com/pod-product-compliance
Lightning Source LLC
Chambersburg PA
CBHW032145020426

42334CB00016B/1238